A Bedside Guide to Mechanical Ventilation

Kenneth Nugent MD
Eva Nourbakhsh MD

D1365371

A Bedside Guide to Mechanical Ventilation
First edition
April 16, 2011

ISBN-10 : 1461102189
EAN-13: 978-1461102182

Editors

Kenneth Nugent MD
Division Chief: Pulmonary Medicine

Eva Nourbakhsh MD
Internal Medicine Resident

Authors

Jessamy Anderson RN, BSN, CCRN, Reza Anvari MD, Gilbert Berdine MD, Cihan Cevik MD, Hugh Frederick Pharm D, Rahul Mishra DO, Eva Nourbakhsh MD, Kenneth Nugent MD, Rishi Raj MD, Rosemary Salazar RRT

Texas Tech University Health Sciences Center, Lubbock
Department of Internal Medicine, Division of Pulmonary Critical Care Medicine
3601 4th Street Stop 9410, Lubbock TX 79416
Phone: (806)743-3155. Fax (806)743-3148.

Acknowledgments

We thank Connie Nugent for editorial assistance and advice on design and page layout.

DISCLAIMER

THIS HANDBOOK IS INTENDED FOR INFORMATION AND REFERENCE USE ONLY.
The information provided is designed to help residents and other health care practitioners understand basic concepts about mechanical ventilation. It is not intended as a substitute for mechanical ventilation textbooks, clinical experience, or clinical judgment. Sources used for this handbook are believed to be reliable and accurate. Efforts were made to include the latest evidence-based recommendations. However, the accuracy and completeness of the information cannot be guaranteed. Therefore, this handbook should be used as a guide and **NOT** as the only source of information for individual patient care. This handbook is sold "as is" without warranties of any kind, express or implied, and all involved with creation and publication of this handbook disclaim any liability, loss, or damages which may arise therefrom.

Contents

Chapter 1 **Key ideas**

1. Most patients who require mechanical ventilation do well with the assist-control mode.

2. Patients with acute lung injury and acute respiratory distress syndrome have better outcomes with a low tidal volume, low plateau pressure ventilation strategy.

3. Nurses should keep the head of the bed elevated and monitor gastric residuals. These precautions reduce the frequency of ventilator-associated pneumonia.

4. Combinations of benzodiazepines and narcotics probably provide optimal patient comfort during mechanical ventilation. Nurses should use a standardized scoring system to titrate the patient's response to sedation protocols. Physicians and nurses should make frequent efforts to wean sedation, and it should be interrupted daily.

5. Physicians and respiratory therapists should make frequent efforts to reduce FiO_2 and should use the ARDS Network Table for FiO_2 and PEEP combinations.

6. The initial treatment for ventilator-associated pneumonia should provide broad spectrum antibiotic coverage for multidrug resistant hospital-acquired pathogens. De-escalation of this therapy is appropriate when cultures results are available.

7. Physicians should review the patient's weaning potential daily. Spontaneous breathing trials and weaning parameters help make optimal decisions about extubation.

8. Immediate physiologic changes do not always reflect long term benefit or harm for the patient. The clinician should be flexible and at times allow pH to be lower or CO_2 to be higher. Clinical judgment is important.

Study question

Based on your reading or your clinical experience list three ideas which are likely important in the care of **every** patient on a mechanical ventilator.

Chapter 2 **Respiratory physiology**

Respiratory Drive Controllers

Central chemoreceptors
- Located in the medulla.
- Respond to changes in pH of CSF.
- Mechanism: $\uparrow CO_2$ in arterial blood $\rightarrow$ crosses the blood brain barrier $\rightarrow$ in CSF, CO_2 combines with H_2O $\rightarrow$ produces $H^+ + HCO_3^-$.
- $\uparrow H^+$ acts in central chemoreceptors causing hyperventilation via vagus nerve stimulation.
- $\downarrow$ CSF pH causes hyperventilation which decreases CO_2 in blood.

Peripheral chemoreceptors
- They are located at bifurcation of common carotid arteries above and below the aortic arch. They act through three different mechanisms.
- $\downarrow$ arterial pO_2 (<60 mm Hg) $\rightarrow$ activation of chemoreceptors $\rightarrow$ **hyperventilation.**
- $\uparrow$ arterial $pO_2 \rightarrow$ partial inactivation of chemoreceptors $\rightarrow$ normal ventilation.
- $\uparrow$ arterial $H^+ \rightarrow$ activation of carotid bodies at bifurcation $\rightarrow$ **hyperventilation** to correct pH.

Lung stretch receptors
- Located in smooth muscles of airways.
- Stimulated by lung distention $\rightarrow$ slows inspiration (Hering- Breurer reflex).

Irritant receptors
- Located between epithelial cells of airways.
- Stimulated by particulates.
- Cause reflex bronchoconstriction $\rightarrow$ coughing and $\uparrow$ RR.

Juxtacapillary receptors
- Located in alveolar walls next to capillaries.
- Any change in size of these capillaries causes activation of these receptors, e.g., pulmonary edema.
- Cause $\uparrow$ RR.

Gas Exchange

Hypoxemia

- $\downarrow PO_2$ caused by $\downarrow$ inspired O_2, hypoventilation, diffusion defects, ventilation to perfusion ($\dot{V}/\dot{Q}$) mismatch, and R to L shunt.
- The degree of hypoxemia can be calculated by using A-a gradient, which is the difference between alveolar oxygen pressure (PAO_2) and arterial oxygen pressure (PaO_2).

    A-a gradient = PAO_2 – PaO_2

    Equation:
    $PAO_2 = PiO_2 - PACO_2/R$
    $PiO_2 = FiO_2 (Patm - 47mmHg) \rightarrow 0.21(760 - 47) \rightarrow 0.21(713) \rightarrow$ 150 mmHg
    $PAO_2 = 150$ mmHg $- (PACO_2 \times 1.25)$ mmHg
    Where PiO_2 is inspired oxygen pressure, $PACO_2$ is alveolar CO_2 pressure ($PACO_2 = PaCO_2$), **R** is respiratory exchange ratio (R $\approx$ 0.8) and **Patm** is the atmospheric pressure (760 mmHg at sea level).
    PaO_2 is taken from the ABG result

- Normal A-a gradient is <10 mmHg
- Abnormal A-a gradient is >10mmHg
- An abnormal gradient indicates that gas exchange in the alveolar-capillary unit is abnormal.
- Hypoxemia with normal gradient: $\downarrow$ inspired O_2, hypoventilation.
- Hypoxemia with abnormal gradient:

    - **Diffusion impairment**- increased diffusion distances such as thick basement membranes
    - $\dot{V}/\dot{Q}$ **mismatch** – reduced alveolar ventilation in relationship to perfusion. Diseases include emphysema, bronchitis, asthma, interstitial lung disease.
    - **Shunts** – Alveoli collapse or alveolar filling with exudates, fluid or blood or true anatomic shunt. Examples include ARDS, CHF, hemorrhage, atelectasis, lobar pneumonia.

- To differentiate between $\dot{V}/\dot{Q}$ mismatch and shunt, place patient on supplemental oxygen. With $\dot{V}/\dot{Q}$ mismatch the PaO_2 increases; with R to L shunt there is no change in PaO_2. Patients with diffusion defects usually have hypoxemia during periods of increased cardiac output.

Hypoxemic Respiratory failure (PaO_2 < 55 mm Hg or SaO_2 <88%):
- Decreased inspired PO_2
  - Low PiO_2 at high altitudes
  - Low PiO_2 in fires
- Diffusion limitation
- Ventilation perfusion abnormalities
  - Emphysema
  - Bronchitis
  - Asthma
  - Interstitial lung disease
- Intra-cardiac or intra-pulmonary anatomic shunts
  - Pulmonary embolism
  - Pneumonia
  - Heart Failure
  - ARDS
  - Atelectasis
  - Hemorrhage

Hypercapnia
- ↑ PCO_2 secondary to inadequate alveolar ventilation
- Causes
  - Decreased minute ventilation associated with neuromuscular disease, normal A-a O_2 gradient.
  - Abnormal $\dot{V}/\dot{Q}$ relation associated with parenchymal lung disease, abnormal A-a O_2 gradient.
  - Rarely increased CO_2 production with a fixed minute ventilation.

Hypercapneic respiratory failure ($PaCO_2$ > 50 mmHg):
- COPD
- Asthma
- CNS infection or neoplasm
- Airway obstruction
- Paralysis of the diaphragm due to neurologic disorders
- Effect of anesthetic and muscle relaxant drugs

Lung Mechanics

Airway Resistance

Can be calculated by Ohm's law or Poiseuille's law.

Ohm's law- $R = \Delta P / \dot{V}$

ΔP = Pressure in the mouth – Pressure in alveoli

$\dot{V}$ = Airflow

Poiseuille's law- $R = 8\eta l / \pi r^4$

R= resistance

η = viscosity of inspired gas

l= length of airway

r= radius of airway

As diameter decreases→ resistance increases

Factors that change the resistance:
- Asthma
- Irritants
- Parasympathetic stimulation→↓radius and ↑R
- Sympathetic stimulation→ ↑radius and ↓R
- High lung volume→↑traction of airways→↓R
- Low lung volume→↓traction of airways→↑R
- Viscosity of inspired gas (η):
  - Diving in deep sea→↑η→↑R
  - Helium →↓η→ ↓R.

Compliance of lungs

- $C = \Delta V / \Delta P$ where ΔV is volume change (tidal volume) and ΔP is change in pressure.
- It is a change in volume for a given change in pressure.
- It depends on the amount of elastic tissue in the lungs.
- It depends on transpulmonary pressure which is [alveolar pressure – intrapleural pressure].
- Intrapleural pressure is the pressure outside of the lungs in the pleural space.
- Compliance is greatest when the elasticity of lungs and chest wall is equal.
- Changes in compliance can occur in respiratory diseases such as emphysema (↑compliance) and pulmonary fibrosis (↓compliance) and in chest wall disease such as kyphoscoliosis and pleural effusion

6

Respiratory Muscles
- Muscles used for **inspiration** – diaphragm, external intercostals, and accessory muscles of chest.
- Muscles used for **expiration** – normally is passive as lungs return to end tidal volume, but in exercise or disease, abdominal muscles and internal intercostals muscle can contribute to exhalation.

Ventilation

Information from peripheral and central chemoreceptors produces central respiratory drive. This signal is sent to the diaphragm through the phrenic nerves. When the muscles of respiration contract, the intrapleural pressure becomes more negative causing the lungs to expand and open the alveoli. This causes the pressure in the alveoli to fall below atmospheric pressure and air to flow into the alveoli. Exhalation occurs passively. The net alveolar ventilation maintains a normal $PaCO_2$ and PaO_2.

Study questions

Patients with pleural effusions have decreased chest wall compliance. What happens to airway pressures during positive pressure ventilation of these patients?

Patients with ascites have decreased chest wall compliance. What happens to airway pressures during positive pressure ventilation of patients with significant ascites? What happens to transpulmonary pressure?

Does the abdominal compartment syndrome change peak pressures in patients on ventilators?

Chapter 3 Oxygen therapy

Oxygen therapy can increase PaO_2, O_2 content, and O_2 delivery

Indications
- Acute respiratory distress with hypoxemia
  $PaO_2 \leq 50$ mmHg or $SaO_2 \leq 88\%$

- Chronic hypoxemia with $PaO_2 \leq 55$mmHg

Delivery Methods

Device	Oxygen flow rate (l/min)	FiO$_2$* (%)
Nasal cannula	1	24
	2	28
	3	32
	4	36
	5	40
Face mask	5	40
	6-7	50
	7-8	60
Partial rebreather (w/o side flap)	12-15	70
Non-rebreather	12-15	>90
Venturi mask**	3-15	24-50
Endotracheal tube		21-100

*FiO$_2$ values are approximations. **The color of the adapter reflects the delivered oxygen concentration: Colors (Hudson RCI) 4%:blue; 28%:yellow; 31%:white; 35%:green; 40%:pink; 50%:orange.

Monitoring Goals
- $SaO_2 \geq 88\%$ (measured with pulse oximetry)

- $PaO_2 \geq 55 - 60$ mmHg (measured with ABG)

Estimating PaO_2 from a given SaO_2

SaO$_2$ (%)	80	82	84	86	88	90	92	93	94	95	96	97	98	99
PaO$_2$(mmHg)	44	46	49	52	55	60	65	69	73	79	86	96	112	145

Potential concerns
- High concentrations (FiO$_2 \geq 50\%$) - O_2 toxicity (looks like ARDS)

- COPD and low flow O_2 - CO_2 retention with decreased pH

Study question

How does an increase in the partial pressure of oxygen in the alveolar spaces influence gas exchange?

List beneficial effects.

List potential adverse effects.

Clinical syndromes

- **Failure of the ventilator pump**
  - Alveolar hypoventilation with hypercapnea and hypoxemia
  - Respiratory and neuromuscular disease, including coma and OD
- **Inadequate pulmonary gas exchange**
  - Acute respiratory distress
  - Clinical deterioration, especially shock
  - RR ≥ 35 breaths /min
  - Increased work of breathing→respiratory muscle fatigue
  - Abnormal ABGs

Therapeutic
- CO intoxication
- CNS disease with high intracranial pressure

Inability to protect airways from aspiration
- ↓LOC – Glasgow Coma Scale ≤ 8
- Vocal cord dysfunction

Clinical manifestations of respiratory distress
- Nasal flaring
- Accessory muscle recruitment
- Tracheal tug
- Intercostal recession
- Tachypnea
- Tachycardia
- Hypertension or hypotension
- Diaphoresis
- Changes in mental status

Laboratory evidence of impaired gas exchange
- $PaCO_2 > 50$ mmHg with academia (pH ≤7.25)
- $PaCO_2$ ↑ of 5-10 mmHg from baseline in patients with COPD and a change in clinical status
- $PaO_2 < 55$ mmHg on a $FiO_2 = 60\%$

Goals
- Improve oxygenation
- Increase CO_2 excretion
- Reduce work of breathing

Discussion

Not all the patients with the above indications need ventilator support. There is no threshold of PaO_2 or $PaCO_2$ for which mechanical ventilation is mandatory. The indications are flexible and lack boundaries. Physician judgment is imperative. Because mechanical ventilation only provides assistance for breathing and does not cure disease, it is not indicated if the underlying problem is not correctable.

Study question

Summarize the treatment of the most recent patient you cared for who required mechanical ventilation. What was the indication for mechanical ventilation? Did this decision depend on quantitative information from blood gases or clinical information from bedside assessment?

Chapter 5 **Ventilator basics**

Mechanical ventilation is a method of inspiratory assistance. Ventilators generate and regulate the flow of gas into the lungs until a preset pressure or volume has been generated. Expiration is passive. There are several concepts to understand before ordering mechanical ventilation. Some terms may vary from ventilator to ventilator.

Important considerations when ordering mechanical ventilation

- What control variable do you want- pressure, volume, or both?
- What will be the trigger?
- What mode of ventilator do you want? CMV, AC, SIMV, PC, PRVC, PSV, or APRV
- Do you want spontaneous breaths to be assisted?

Control

A ventilator may be classified as pressure, volume, flow, or time controlled. Some combine control schemes to create complex modes. The conventional modes of mechanical ventilation control either pressure or volume. This variable will remain constant during each breath delivery regardless of changes in lung mechanics.

- **Pressure** control means the pressure is constant and volume is variable.
- **Volume** control means the volume is constant and the pressure is variable.

Cycle

It is the period of time between the beginning of one breath and the beginning of the next.

Trigger

The initiation of a cycle occurs when certain preset variables are reached. The preset value is also known as the trigger.

- **Time**: the ventilator initiates a breath according to a set time.
- **Pressure**: the ventilator senses the patient's inspiratory effort in the form of decrease in baseline pressure and starts inspiration.
- **Flow**: the ventilator senses the inspiratory effort as a decrease in baseline flow through the patient circuit or senses inspiratory flow at the patient's airway opening and starts a breath.
- **Volume**: The ventilator senses a volume change. This is not used frequently in adults.

13

Waveforms

When looking at most mechanical ventilator screens you will notice three different waveforms. One will be for pressure, one for volume, and one for flow. When these values are plotted as functions of time, characteristic waveforms are produced. Waveforms are important for interpretation of bedside lung mechanics. For example, you can detect auto-PEEP from a flow or pressure waveform, or you can detect a leak on the ventilator circuit from the volume waveform.

The waveforms will change depending on the control variable. For example, if the control variable is pressure, the shape of the volume and flow waveforms will depend on the shape of the pressure waveform and on the resistance and compliance of the respiratory system. Waveforms:

- Rectangular (pressure, flow)
- Exponential (pressure)
- Ramp (volume, flow)
- Sinusoidal (pressure, volume)

Shapes of waveforms

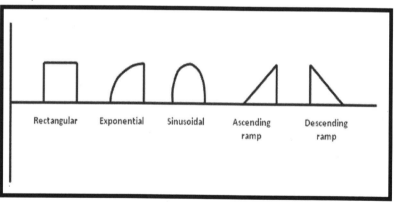

Normal waveforms on ventilator screen

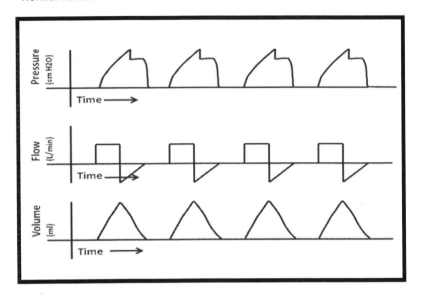

Example of an abnormal waveform

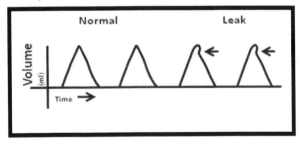

Add Notes or Questions

Chapter 6 Ventilator display and functions

There are over 50 models of adult, ICU, invasive mechanical ventilators. The modes, waveforms, operating range of controls (TV, RR, peak flow, pressure support, PEEP, etc), graphic display, and size vary from model to model. Despite these differences, the purpose remains the same, and clinicians should know standard parameters and measurements. The following measurements are commonly seen on the ventilator screen:

Peak pressure represents the highest pressure needed to move a volume of gas into the lung.
- It reflects the highest pressure applied to major airways during inspiration.
- It can help monitor airway patency.
- Peak pressure will increase with: asthma, mucus plugs, ET tube obstruction.
- High peak pressures increase the risk of barotrauma.
- Peak pressure should not exceed **40 cm H_2O**.
- For example, if a patient's ET tube accidentally moves into one of the main stem bronchi, the peak pressure will increase.

Inspiratory plateau pressure reflects the pressure at end inspiration during a period of no airflow.
- It reflects the pressure applied to small airways and alveoli.
- Used to assess lung compliance: ↓compliance ("stiff lung") → ↑plateau pressure; ↑compliance → ↓plateau pressure.
- High plateau pressure increases the risk of barotrauma.
- Low plateau pressure can result in atelectasis and hypoventilation.
- Plateau pressure should not exceed **30 cm H_2O**.
- For example, patients with ARDS, pulmonary fibrosis, or abdominal distension will have ↑ plateau pressure.

Mean airway pressure (Pmean) is the average pressure throughout the ventilatory cycle.
- This incorporates all pressures to which the lungs are exposed during the respiratory cycle.
- The mean airway pressure will increase if the PEEP is increased.
- Trends in Pmean may provide useful information.
- Monitored in patients on APRV or high frequency ventilation.
- ↑ in ARDS; ↓in emphysema.

Positive end-expiratory pressure (PEEP) is externally applied pressure that maintains a positive airway pressure throughout expiration
- Please refer to PEEP chapter (9).

Inspiratory time (Ti) is the time between the start of inspiration and the start of exhalation.
- Longer inspiratory time is associated with improved oxygenation but increases the risk of auto-PEEP.

Expiratory time (Te) is the time between the start of expiration and the start of inspiration.

I: E ratio is the ratio between inspiratory time and expiratory time.
- Usual ratio is 1:2 to 1:3

Minute volume ($\dot{V}_E$) is the amount of gas moved in and out of the respiratory system in one minute
- Tidal volume multiplied by respiratory rate.
- The higher the $\dot{V}_E$ the more CO_2 is excreted.
- The normal $\dot{V}_E$ is 5-8 L/min.
- $\uparrow \dot{V}_E$ may reflect inefficient gas exchange or hyperventilation.
- $\downarrow \dot{V}_E$ may cause hypoxemia or hypercapnia.
- For example, patients with ARDS often have an increased $\dot{V}_E$.

Inspiratory minute volume (MV_{IN}) is the volume delivered in one minute during inspiration.
- This number is patient dependent on some modes of ventilation.

Expiratory minute volume (MV_{EX}) is the exhaled volume in one minute.
- MV_{IN} and MV_{EX} should be the same.
- Please refer to troubleshooting chapter.

Inspiratory tidal volume (V_{TI}) is the tidal volume during inspiration.
- A small V_T can result in hypoxemia, atelectasis, or hypoventilation.
- A large V_T can result in hyperventilation, volutrauma, or low CO_2.

Expiratory tidal volume (V_{TE}) is the tidal volume during exhalation.
- V_{TI} and V_{TE} should be the same.
- Please refer to troubleshooting chapter (23).

Cuff Pressures
- Endotracheal tubes (ETT) have a cuff to seal the airway. The pressure used to inflate the cuff can be measured with a manometer.
- The cuff pressure should be kept < 20 mmHg. The cuff pressure should not exceed 25 mmHg; this should limit pressure induced necrosis.
- High cuff pressures cause physical trauma to the trachea and/or impede blood flow to the tracheal mucosa.
- Measured once a shift by RT.

Lung compliance is the measurement of the distensibility of the lung.
- **Static compliance** measures the elastic properties of the lung.
  - ↓ static compliance may be due to pleural or chest wall disorders .
- **Dynamic compliance** measures both elastic and resistive forces.
  - ↓ dynamic compliance may be due to ↑ resistance, such as with excessive secretions, bronchospasm, occlusion of ETT, or a kink in tubing.
- ↓ in both dynamic and the static compliance may be caused by atelectasis, pneumothorax, pulmonary edema, ARDS, mainstem intubation, or worsening of the underlying disorder.
  - Formulas:
    ### Static Compliance
    V_{TE} / (Plateau pressure – PEEP)
    Normal value **>60 ml/cmH$_2$0**
    ### Dynamic Compliance
    V_{TE} / (Peak pressure – PEEP)
    Normal range **40-50 ml/cmH$_2$O**
- **Clinical relevance**
  ↓ Compliance secondary to **lung** problems
    - Worsening ARDS
    - Pneumonia
    - Pulmonary edema
  ↓ Compliance secondary to **chest wall/pleural** problems
    - Pneumothorax (MOST IMPORTANT)
    - Pleural fluid collections (pleural effusions, hemothorax)
    - Decreased chest wall compliance (extreme obesity, scarring post burns, etc.)
  ↓ Compliance secondary to **Non-thoracic** problems
    - Severe abdominal distension (massive ascites, abdominal compartment syndrome, etc.)

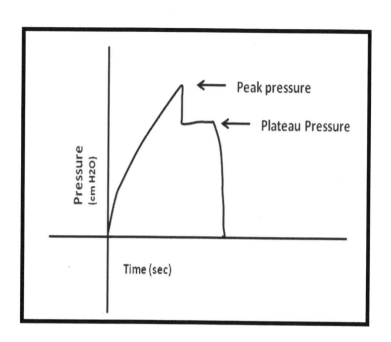

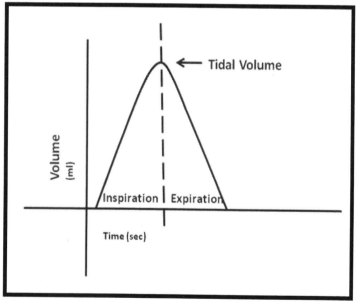

Chapter 7 **Modes of ventilation**

Ventilator modes

The key differences between ventilator modes include the trigger (what initiates the inspiratory phase), the cycle length (what terminates the inspiratory phase), and the primary output (a preset tidal volume or a preset pressure). Other important factors include safety limits set by the operator and patient interaction with the ventilator.

CMV - Continuous mandatory ventilation

The ventilator delivers a preset tidal volume at a preset rate. The patient cannot trigger the breath. This mode is frequently used in paralyzed patients and during general anesthesia with the use of muscle relaxants. The assist/control mode defaults to this mode when the patient does not trigger the ventilator.

Preset
- Tidal volume
- RR
- FiO_2
- PEEP

AC - Assist/control ventilation

The ventilator delivers a preset tidal volume during every inspiration. The breath can be triggered either by the ventilator at a preset back-up rate or by the patient at his/her spontaneous respiratory rate. The mandatory breath occurs at a preset time after the previous inspiration if the patient does not trigger the machine. This is the most commonly used mode.

Preset
- Tidal volume
- RR
- FiO_2
- PEEP

SIMV - Synchronized intermittent mandatory ventilation

This is a combination mode in which the patient receives mandatory breaths synchronized with his/her respiratory effort and can take spontaneous breaths between the mandatory breaths. The cycle can be divided in two phases, the SIMV phase and the spontaneous phase. During the SIMV phase any triggered breath results in a preset tidal volume. If the patient has not triggered a breath within the first 90% of the SIMV phase, a mandatory breath is delivered. During the spontaneous phase the patient cannot trigger the ventilator and the tidal volume delivered, if any,

21

depends on the patient's effort. These spontaneous breaths can be pressure supported. This mode is often used as a weaning mode by decreasing the SIMV phase and allowing the patient to take more spontaneous breaths.

Preset
- Tidal volume
- RR
- FiO$_2$
- PEEP

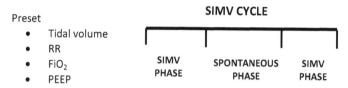

SIMV CYCLE

| SIMV PHASE | SPONTANEOUS PHASE | SIMV PHASE |

PC - Pressure control

The ventilator delivers the same pressure during every inspiration, and this pressure is maintained throughout the inspiratory cycle. The resulting tidal volume depends on the set pressure level, the inspiratory time, and the patient's lung mechanics. The mandatory breath occurs at a preset frequency or when triggered by the patient. Expiration starts after termination of the inspiratory time or when the upper pressure limit is exceeded.

Preset
- Pressure
- RR
- FiO$_2$
- PEEP

PRVC - Pressure regulated volume control

This mode combines the advantages of volume controlled and pressure controlled ventilation. The ventilator delivers a preset tidal volume at a constant pressure which continuously adapts to the patient's lung mechanics. The preset tidal volume occurs at a preset frequency or when the patient triggers the ventilator. Expiration occurs at the end of inspiration or when the upper pressure limit is exceeded. The delivered tidal volumes can be higher than the preset tidal volumes.

Preset
- Tidal volume
- RR
- V$_T$
- FiO$_2$
- PEEP
- Upper pressure limit (not >40 cm H$_2$O)

22

PSV - Pressure support ventilation

The patient's inspiratory effort is assisted by the ventilator to a preset level of inspiratory pressure. The patient determines the frequency, inspiratory time, and tidal volume. Therefore the minute ventilation depends on the underlying respiratory drive and lung mechanics. Some mechanical ventilators have a backup apnea rate when using this mode.

Preset
- Pressure
- FiO_2
- PEEP

Patient controls
- RR
- Flow rate
- V_T

APRV - explained in Chapter 11

Common parameters practice

V_T (for volume control)
- When writing for V_T it is important to calculate IBW first.
- Maximum V_T 10 mL/kg IBW in patients without lung disease.
- <10 mL/kg IBW in patients with lung disease.
- 6 ml/kg IBW in ALI/ARDS.

Pressure (for pressure control)
- Start with 20-25 cm H_2O.
- ↑ or ↓ about 5 cm H_2O.
- Adjust to maintain VT 6-8 mL/kg IBW.

RR
- Start 12-16 breath per minute.
- 18-22 breaths per minute in patients with ALI/ARDS.
- ↑ or ↓ 1-2 breaths per minute.

FiO_2
- Start with FiO_2 100%.
- Adjust FiO_2 for a goal $SaO_2 \geq 88\%$ or $PaO_2 \geq 55$ mmHg.
- ↑ or ↓ by 0.5-.10 increments.

PEEP
- Start with a PEEP of 5cm H_2O.
- ↑ PEEP by 2-3cm H_2O every 30-60 minutes.
- Refer to PEEP chapter for ARDS table.

Inspiratory time
- Start with 0.8-1 sec.
- Adjustments are infrequent unless auto-PEEP is present.

I: E ratio
- Start with 1:2.
- Adjust to 1:3, 1:4.
- May change ratio as well, for example to 2:1 or 3:1.

Flow
- It can be adjusted on some ventilators.
- Range 30-60 L/min.
- Patients with COPD may need higher flows for "air hunger".
- ↓ the inspiratory time will ↑ the flow.

Monitor

- Peak pressure
- Plateau pressure
- Waveform
- I: E ratio
- Flow rate

Adjustments

- FiO_2
- Trigger sensitivity
- Backup rate
- Tidal volume
- Inspiratory flow rate (or inspired time)
- End inspiratory pause
- External PEEP

Immediate Goals

- Stabilize the patient.
- Promote adequate oxygenation.
- Maintain patient comfort.
- Adjust ventilator to maintain the patient's "usual" PCO_2.
- To improve oxygenation: ↑ FiO_2 and/or PEEP
- To increase ventilation (↓CO_2): ↑ RR or ↑V_T
- Also refer to troubleshooting chapters (22 and 23)

Case analysis

Write down the machine parameters used on the last patient you cared for who had acute respiratory failure. In retrospect, were these good choices? Were you satisfied with the resulting gas exchange?

Mode	A/C
Tidal Volume	Calculate IBW IBW x 6-8 ml will give you the V_T
RR	12-14 breaths per minute
FiO$_2$	100%
PEEP	5 cm H$_2$0
Order	STAT CXR for ET tube for placement ABG 30-60 minutes post intubation
Start sedation and pain control if needed	**Sedation** Midazolam: Start at 0.04-0.2 mg/kg/hour and titrate to RASS scale of -1 to -2. **Pain** Fentanyl: 0.7-10 mcg/kg/hour, titrate for pain/agitation control.
	Evaluate your patient

Study question

Which ventilator parameters influence $PaCO_2$ the most?

Which ventilator parameters influence PaO_2 the most?

Chapter 9 Use of positive end-expiratory pressure (PEEP)

PEEP is a set on a mechanical ventilator. It is the airway pressure at the end of expiration that is above atmospheric pressure. The main purpose is to prevent small airway collapse at the end of expiration and improve oxygenation. The usual range is 5-25 cmH_2O.

Goal: To use a level of PEEP that allows for the lowest FiO_2 while maintaining adequate oxygenation and avoiding adverse effects

Indications
- ALI/ARDS
- Multilobar pneumonia
- Pulmonary edema
- Atelectasis
- Other forms of hypoxemic respiratory failure

Contraindications
- Increased intracranial pressure
- Pneumothorax without pleural catheter
- Bronchopleural fistula
- Untreated hypovolemia
- Low cardiac output
- Recent pulmonary resection

Positive Effects
- Improves alveolar recruitment
- ↑ Functional residual capacity
- Improves gas exchange and oxygenation
- Redistributes fluid in alveoli
- ↓ FiO_2 requirement
- Helps prevent alveolar collapse
- Improves lung compliance
- Minimizes ventilator-induced lung injury

Negative Effects
- Can worsen gas exchange
- Decreases venous return and preload
- Decreases cardiac output (CO)
- Can cause hypotension and organ hypoperfusion
- Can cause barotrauma
- Can increase intracranial pressure (ICP)

PEEP in practice
- Start with a PEEP of 5cm H_2O
- ↑ PEEP by 2-3cm H_2O every 30-60 minutes to achieve SaO_2 > 88% or PaO_2 > 55 mm Hg
- Refer to ARDS Net table for combination recommendations
- Call for help if you reach a PEEP of 15 and there is no improvement

ARDS Net original PEEP/ FiO_2 combination recommendation

FiO_2	0.3	0.4	.04	0.5	0.5	0.6	0.7	0.7	0.7	0.8	0.9	0.9	0.9	1.0
PEEP	5	5	8	8	10	10	10	12	14	14	14	16	18	18-24

Monitor:

- PaO_2 or SaO_2
- Vital signs ($\downarrow$venous return $\rightarrow$hypotension)
- Level of consciousness ($\downarrow$CO or $\uparrow$ ICP may cause $\downarrow$LOC)
- Organ hypoperfusion (examples, $\downarrow$urine output, $\downarrow$LOC, $\uparrow$lactate)
- Barotrauma (pneumothorax, subcutaneous emphysema)
- Plateau pressure (< 30 cmH$_2$O is good, >35 cmH$_2$O is bad)

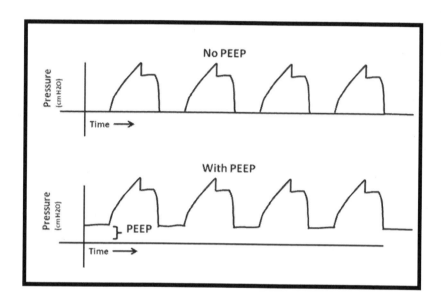

Study question

Patients with ARDS do not have uniform lung involvement. How might PEEP have beneficial effects in some regions of the lung? How might PEEP have deleterious effects in some regions of the lung?

Chapter 10 **Auto-PEEP**

Auto-PEEP occurs in patients on mechanical ventilation when inspiration occurs prior to the end of expiration. The alveolar emptying is incomplete, and the alveolar pressure will be positive in relation to atmospheric pressure. Other terms used are intrinsic PEEP, air trapping, or dynamic hyperinflation.

Causes
- Disease-associated
    o Asthma, COPD, ARDS, bronchospasm, trauma
- Ventilation-associated
    o High inflation volumes ($\uparrow V_T$)
    o High minute ventilation ($\uparrow$RR)
    o Decreased exhalation time relative to inhalation time ($\uparrow$I:E ratio)
    o Anything blocking the exhalation system of the ventilator

Negative Effects

- Decreases venous return and preload
- Decreases cardiac output (CO)
- Causes hypotension and organ hypoperfusion
- Shifts $\dot{V}/\dot{Q}$ relationships and may worsen gas exchange
- Increases intracranial pressure (ICP)
- Causes barotrauma

How to diagnose

- Pressure waveform – the waveform starts at a higher level
- Flow waveform - a breath is initiated before complete exhalation, before reaching baseline
- On the monitor you will notice two PEEP values: the set PEEP and the patient's PEEP. The patient's PEEP> the set PEEP.

What to do
- Review waveforms and measure end-expiratory pressure
- Increase bronchodilator therapy in patients with airway disease
- Prolong expiratory time (example, change I:E ratio 1:2$\rightarrow$1:3)
- Decrease RR
- Decrease minute ventilation by making patient more comfortable
- Review sedation
- Consider permissive hypercapnia

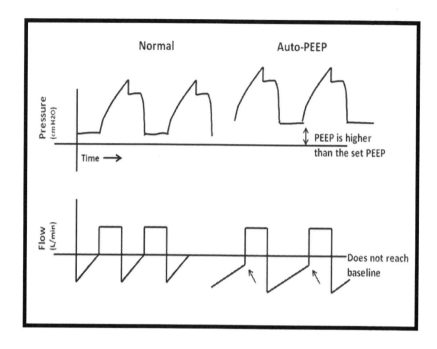

Normal   Auto-PEEP

Pressure (cmH2O)

Time →

PEEP is higher than the set PEEP

Flow (L/min)

Does not reach baseline

Study question

A patient with severe COPD requires intubation of mechanical ventilation. Shortly after mechanical ventilation is started he has a significant decrease in blood pressure. List three possible causes for this situation. List a possible treatment for each of these causes.

Chapter 11 Airway pressure release ventilation (APRV)

This mode is often described as two levels of CPAP that are applied for set periods of time, allowing spontaneous breathing to occur at both levels. The clinician sets the two CPAP levels (pressure high and pressure low) and the time spent at each level (time high and time low).

Physiology/general principles

- APRV is a form of pressure controlled ventilation.
- It delivers inverse ratio ventilation (the inspiration is longer than the expiration).
  - Example of common I:E ratio setting: APRV 4:1 vs. AC 1:2
- It will increase mean airway pressure (Pmean) without increasing peak pressures.
- It allows for superimposed spontaneous ventilation by the patient.
- There is no respiratory rate on APRV; the cycles are measured as "releases" per minute.

When to use this mode of ventilation

- Patients with non-obstructive pulmonary physiology (ARDS) who are difficult to oxygenate using conventional modes. (Reference 1,2)
  - Example, a patient with ARDS on AC on FiO_2 100%, PEEP 15-20

Parameters and what they mean

- P-High: it is the upper pressure. The airway stays at this level for most of the cycle.
  - The higher the P-High, the higher the risk of barotrauma
  - ↑ P-High will ↑ V_T → better oxygenation
  - ↓ P-High will ↓ V_T → worse oxygenation

- P-Low: it is the setting to which the airway pressure drops intermittently, also known as "airway release".
  - ↑P-low will ↓ V_T
  - ↓P-Low will ↑ V_T

- T-High: this is the time spent during P-High.
  - The longer the T-High the longer the alveoli stay open.
  - The longer the T-High the better oxygenation.
  - ↑ T-High will ↓ frequency of "releases" per minute →↑ PCO_2
  - ↓ T-High will ↑ frequency of "releases" per minute→ ↓ PCO_2
  - It should be set 8-12 times longer than the T-Low.

- T-Low: is the time spent on P-Low.
    - Alveoli collapse occurs during this time.
    - It should be kept short to avoid de-recruitment.
    - If this time is too long, it will result in worsening oxygenation.
    - If it is too short, it will cause hypercarbia.

- Termination Peak Expiratory Flow Rate (TPEFR): It is an expiratory flow rate termination point.
    - Used to determine the optimal duration of T-Low
    - Expiration is terminated early in order to create an auto-PEEP and keep the alveoli open.
    - Experts have recommended allowing an expiration of 50% - 75% of normal.
    - ↓T- low will bring TPERF closer to 75% and will improve hypoxemia.
    - ↑T-low will bring TPEFR closer to 50% and will improve hypercarbia.

Initial Settings

- Pressure
    - P-High: 20 cmH$_2$O to keep V$_T$ 6-8ml/kg IBW
    - P-Low: 0 cmH$_2$O
- Time
    - T-High: 4 seconds
    - T-Low :0.7 seconds
- FiO$_2$
    - 100%

Parameter to monitor

- Tidal volume: this is a dependent variable; the operator does not set it. Since most of the patients on APRV have ARDS, aim for 6ml/kg IBW.
- TPEFR: keep between 50-75%. Do not change if PCO$_2$ and oxygenation are acceptable

Trouble shooting
- High V_T:
  - ↑ P-Low
- Hypoxic:
  - ↑ P-High by 1-2 cm increments
  - ↑ T-High by 0.5-1 sec increments
  - ↓ T-low to make TPEFR closer to 75% by 0.1 sec decrements
- Hypercapnea:
  - ↓ T-High by 0.5-1 sec decrements
  - ↑ T-Low to make TPEFR closer to 50%
  - Decrease sedation
  - Allow permissive hypercapnea

Avoid
- Paralysis or over sedation of the patient to the point of suppressing his/her ventilator drive
- ↓ P-High to decrease V_T because it will worsen oxygenation
- APRV in patients with significant obstructive airway disease

Weaning
- Patient should be breathing spontaneously.
- Gradually increase the T-High (in 1 sec increments) while progressively decreasing the P-High (in 1 cm decrements) every 4-8hrs according to gas exchange
- Continue until the parameters are acceptable enough for weaning trials

IMPORTANT: *Please seek expert advice when using this mode.*

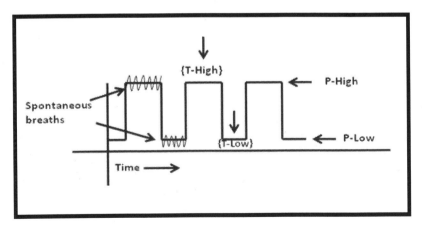

Add Study Notes or Questions

Chapter 12 **Salvage strategies for severe hypoxemia**

Prone positioning
- Reverses atelectasis in dependent lung zones
- Increases PaO_2
- No change in mortality at 28 or 180 days (Ref 3)
- More complications, e.g., tube displacement, skin necrosis

Nitric Oxide
- Bronchodilator and vasodilator effects when inhaled
- Increases PaO_2
- Therapeutic range 5 – 20 ppm
- No change on duration of ventilation or mortality (Ref 4)

High frequency oscillatory ventilation
- High frequency (> 60/min), low tidal volume (1-2 ml/g)
- Volume is 'pushed' into the lung and 'pulled out'
- Mean airway pressure can be high
- No change in mortality (Ref 5)

Corticosteroids
- Limit fibroproliferation and inflammation in ARDS
- No change in mortality at 60 or 180 days (Ref 6, annotated bibliography)

Recruitment maneuver
- High pressure for longer period of inflation, e.g., 40 cm H_2O for 40 seconds
- Usually followed by an increase in PEEP
- Peak effect occurs in 10 minutes, no prolonged effect
- No change in mortality (Ref 6)
- Can decrease the blood pressure and cause barotrauma

IMPORTANT: Please seek expert advice when using these modes

Study question

Patients with refractory hypoxemia present management problems in the ICU. Please consider the various factors that influence oxygen delivery to tissue. List the potential therapeutic interventions which might increase oxygen delivery.

What are the potential side effects of corticosteroids in the acutely ill ICU patient?

Chapter 13 Non-invasive ventilation

Non-invasive ventilation (NIV) is a form of mechanical ventilation using devices that do not require intubation.

Types/Division

- Non-invasive **Positive Pressure** Ventilation (NIPPV)
  - Continuous Positive Airway Pressure (CPAP)
  - Bi-level Positive Airway Pressure (BiPAP)
- Non-invasive **Negative Pressure** Ventilation(NINPV)

NIPPV

It uses a face mask, nasal mask, or helmet mask. It delivers forced air into lungs causing expansion of thoracic cavity and a positive pressure inside the lungs.

CPAP

- The machine delivers the same pressure during inspiration and exhalation.
- It allows pressurized air to splint open the upper airway throughout respiration.
- The pressurized air is titrated (cm H_2O) according to the patient's response.
- CPAP machines can deliver pressure from 4 to 30 cm H_2O.
- It uses a mask that covers either the nose or both the nose and mouth.
- It is most commonly used in obstructive sleep apnea.

BiPAP

- The machine delivers different pressures in inspiration and expiration.
- The inspiratory positive airway pressure is higher than the expiratory positive airway pressure and supports the work of breathing.

Indications in ICU

- COPD, acute exacerbation
- Acute pulmonary edema
- Acute respiratory failure in immunocompromised patient
- Decompensated obstructive sleep apnea
- Pneumonia

Contraindications

- Severe facial trauma or burns
- Severe epistaxis
- CSF leak
- Unconscious patients
- Seizure
- Stroke
- Increased ICP
- Cardiac arrest
- Vomiting
- Upper GI bleed
- Recent stomach surgery
- Systolic pressure < 90
- Risk of aspiration
- Penetrating chest trauma
- Pneumothorax
- Poor compliance
- Increased secretion

Complications

- Excess gas in stomach causing bloating and discomfort
- Nasal congestion
- Increased ear pressure
- Headache
- Skin necrosis

Common parameters in practice

- **Pressure**
  Inhaled – 6 to 12 cmH_2O (IPAP)
  Exhaled – 3 to 6 cmH_2O (EPAP)
  Start with pressures **10** (IPAP)/**5**(EPAP)
- **FiO_2**
  100%
- **RR**
  Set by patient
  Back-up rate 8-10 breaths/min on some machines

Monitor

- BP, HR, RR, SaO_2 in the next 5 minutes to see if there is an improvement.
- Usually by 5 minutes patient should have ↓BP, ↓HR, ↓RR, and ↑SaO_2.
- Within a 2 hour period it should be clear whether the patient is responding well to BiPAP or whether he/she will require intubation.

Troubleshooting

- If oxygenation does not improve, ↑ EPAP
- If ventilation is the problem (e.g., ↑CO_2), ↑ IPAP
- Monitor the V_T measured by the machine
- May increase both pressures by 2 cmH_2O every 5 minutes.
- Call for expert advice if pressures >20 cmH_2O are reached.
- Wean FiO_2 to keep SaO_2 >88% or PaO_2>55 mmHg
- May increase back-up rate if needed.

NINPV

Developed by Dalziel in 1832 and modified to create passive expansion of chest wall and lungs by Drinker-Shaw in 1928. It was commonly used in outbreak of poliomyelitis in 1931.The device is a long closed chambered bed with the patient positioned so the patient's head and neck are outside of the chamber. The negative pressure inside the chamber causes the passive expansion of the chest wall and air flow into the lungs. This device is no longer used in ICUs.

Study question

Patients managed with non-invasive positive pressure ventilation do not require endotracheal intubation. This should reduce some complications associated with mechanical ventilation. List those complications.

Chapter 14 **Positive pressure ventilation effects on cardiac function**

The effects of **mechanical ventilation** on the **cardiovascular system** depend on the baseline myocardial reserve, circulating intravascular volume, intrathoracic pressure (ITP), and autonomic tone of the patient. Unlike spontaneous inspiration, ITP increases during positive-pressure ventilation during lung expansion. Increased ITP causes a reduction of right ventricular filling and pulmonary perfusion. The right atrial pressure and systemic venous pressure increase. Venous return to the heart becomes greatest during expiration which is opposite with spontaneous respiration. The consequence of increased ITP and decreased venous return could be deleterious in patients who are hypovolemic at baseline. These patients may require large volume resuscitation to increase their cardiac output. However, in patients whose intravascular volume is normal or increased, positive pressure ventilation does not impair cardiac output as long as hyperinflation is avoided. Hyperinflation compresses the alveolar vessels, increases pulmonary vascular resistance, and can cause pulmonary artery hypertension. The consequence of hyperinflation in any patient on mechanical ventilation could be acute right ventricular ischemia and failure. Increased right ventricular afterload elevates right ventricular end-diastolic pressure which can result in ventricular septal shift toward the left ventricular cavity.

On the other hand, increased ITP reduces left ventricular afterload, which in turn, augments left ventricular systolic function and cardiac output. This beneficial effect is even more pronounced in patients with myocardial ischemia at baseline. Positive pressure ventilation decreases the work of breathing, increases oxygen delivery to other organs, and decreases myocardial oxygen demand. These effects improve myocardial contractility and cardiac output and reduce ischemia. The opposite situation develops during transition from positive pressure ventilation to spontaneous breathing. The weaning from positive pressure ventilation to spontaneous breathing usually represents an

43

acute cardiovascular stress. Therefore, withdrawal of ventilator support in patients with reduced cardiovascular reserve can precipitate myocardial ischemia, heart failure, and pulmonary edema.

The autonomic balance is altered in patients with acute respiratory failure. These patients have elevated catecholamine levels secondary to anxiety, dyspnea, and hypoxia. Mechanical ventilation is useful in protecting the myocardium from the excessive catecholamine release by eliminating dyspnea, anxiety, and maintaining ventilator support. This effect is also beneficial in reducing the dysrhythmias induced by elevated adrenergic tone.

In summary, the effects of positive pressure ventilation on cardiac function are very complex and variable since most of these changes depend on the baseline cardiovascular status of the patient and the etiology of the respiratory compromise. These effects are minimized by using the lowest possible mean airway pressure. The maintenance cardiac output and systemic blood pressure can be achieved by volume repletion with or without vasopressor drugs when a high mean airway pressure is necessary. The most common effects on the cardiovascular system in a usual patient without accompanying significant comorbidities are summarized in the following table.

Positive Pressure Ventilation	Usual Effects on Cardiovascular System	
	Increase	Decrease
Intrathoracic pressure	↑	
Systemic venous pressure	↑	
Right atrial pressure	↑	
Pulmonary artery pressure	↑	
Tricuspid regurgitation	↑	
Inferior vena cava diameter	↑	
Cardiac output		↓
Myocardial oxygen demand		↓
Heart rate		↓
Systemic venous return		↓
Left ventricular afterload		↓
Left ventricular ejection	↑	
Mixed venous oxygen saturation	↑	
PaO$_2$	↑	
Pulmonary vascular resistance	↑	
Right ventricular afterload	↑	
Right ventricular ejection fraction		↓
Right ventricular volumes		↓
Systemic arterial pressure		↓

Table summarizes the most common changes in the cardiovascular system during positive pressure ventilation. These effects vary according to baseline cardiac, pulmonary, and vascular status and the etiology of respiratory insufficiency. Right heart catheterization can provide more information on the cardiovascular status and hemodynamics in some complex patients.

Study question

Patients with acute respiratory failure secondary to cardiogenic pulmonary edema almost always benefit from mechanical ventilation with positive intra-thoracic pressures. List the potential benefits of mechanical ventilation on myocardial function and gas exchange. Will the withdrawal of a positive intra-thoracic pressure have any influence on myocardial function which might delay weaning?

Chapter 15 Comprehensive care of the ventilated patient

Patient Position

- The patient's head should be elevated at least 30 degrees.
- Patients need frequent turning to prevent pressure ulcers on bony prominences.

DVT Prophylaxis

- Prophylactic doses of either low molecular heparin or unfractionated heparin when possible.
- Sequential compression devices in patients who cannot receive heparin products.

Stress Gastritis

- These patients should receive either H_2 blockers or proton pump inhibitors. Enteral feeding can eliminate the need for medication provided the patient has no other co-morbidities which increase the risk of gastric ulceration.

Sedation Management

- All sedation titration should be based on the use of a sedation scoring system, such as the RASS.
- Anxiolytic and narcotic medications should be stopped daily to assess the patient's mental status and the need for continued sedation and/or pain management.

Nutrition

- Patients need 25 to 30 calories per kilogram per day usually supplied by enteral feeding.
- Patients need 1 – 1.5 grams of protein per kilogram per day supplied by enteral feeding.
- Patients need 60 to 100 mEq of potassium per day (caution in patients with renal disease).
- Patients need 60 to 100 mEq of sodium per day.
- Serum glucose level should be kept in the range or 110 to 180 mg/dl.
- Monitor gastric residuals- high volumes >250 ml increase the risk for aspiration.

Add Notes or Questions

Chapter 16 **Daily check list for clinicians**

- **Review the chart for**
  - Acute events overnight
- **Check vital signs**
  - Pulse rate
  - Respiratory rate
  - O_2 saturation
  - Blood pressure
- **Check fluid balance**
- **Examine chest for**
  - Air entry
  - Breath sounds
  - Crackles
  - Wheezing
- **Check endotracheal tube for**
  - Position at mouth/teeth to note significant movement
  - Secretions
- **Check ventilator screen for**
  - PEEP level
  - Peak airway pressure
  - Plateau airway pressure
- **Check ABG**
- **Check chest x-ray for**
  - ET tube position
  - Catheter position
  - Presence of infiltrates
  - Presence of pneumothorax, pneumomediastinum, subcutaneous emphysema
- **Review sedation management and other medications**
  - Assess patient's comfort
  - Adjust sedation to keep RASS between -1 to -2 (Chapter 18)
  - Discontinue sedation every morning
- **Review clinical course**
  - Current FiO_2
  - Trends in FiO_2
  - Weaning potential
- **Make therapeutic and diagnostic decisions**
  - Reduce PEEP as FiO_2 is reduced.
  - Consider spontaneous breathing trial
- **Write new orders** (consider daily X-ray and ABGs on all ventilated patients)

Study Question

Does over sedation have any important effects on patient outcomes? Explain your answer.

Chapter 17 **RT daily duties in the ICU**

The **daily duties** of a respiratory therapist start with receiving report from the RT assigned the previous shift, followed by walking rounds and a ventilator check. The ventilator is checked every 2 hours. Following the initial ventilator check, a ventilator assessment is performed. The ventilator assessment is performed once a shift at the beginning of the shift.

Ventilator setting check includes
- Ventilator mode
- FiO_2
- Set tidal volume
- Ventilator rate
- PEEP
- Inspiratory time
- I:E Ratio
- Flow rate
- Inspiratory pause time

Ventilator parameters check includes
- Peak airway pressure
- Plateau pressure
- Mean airway pressure
- Spontaneous respiratory rate
- Inhaled tidal volume
- Exhaled tidal volume
- Minute volume
- Lung compliance
- Ventilator circuit temperature and humidity
- Filter check

Ventilator assessment includes
- Ambu bag with PEEP valve in place and face mask at bedside for emergent care
- Check alarms that are set and functioning for patient safety
- ETT placement
- Cuff pressures
- Listen to breath sounds
- Suction if needed

Respiratory medication review
- Dose and frequency

Study questions

Look up the "normal" compliance for patients on ventilators. Which patients tend to have a low compliance? Which patients tend to have a high compliance?

Chapter 18 Routine nursing care for ventilator patients

Oral care
- Routine oral assessment every 2-4 hours.
- Brush teeth twice daily.
- Assess lips, oral mucosa, tongue, gums, teeth, and soft and hard palate at least twice daily.
- Oral endotracheal tubes will be retaped and repositioned side to side in the patient's mouth every 24 hours. All endotracheal tubes will be securely taped or tied.
- Oral care for patients who are receiving positive pressure ventilation or who have a tracheostomy should be done according to an oral care policy.

Suctioning
- Use clinical indicators for the need to suction (should not be performed "routinely") and limit the number of passes to minimum required:
    - Tachycardia, tachypnea
    - Change in BP
    - Dyspnea
    - Noisy or shallow ventilation
    - Rhonchi
    - Obvious visible secretions
    - Excessive coughing during inspiratory cycle of ventilator
    - High-pressure alarm on vent
    - Low SaO_2
- Instillation of saline/saline lavage is ineffective and potentially harmful.
- Subglottic suctioning every 8 hours.

Gastric Residuals
- Checked every 4 hours.

Positioning
- Turning every 2 hours.
- Kinetic therapy to promote redistribution of ventilation and perfusion and optimize $\dot{V}/\dot{Q}$ matching.
    - Indicated for ALI, ARDS, pneumonia
- Prone position
    - Consider in ALI, ARDS

Richmond Agitation and Sedation Scale (RASS)

- Sedation is important in ventilated patients. Too little sedation can result in patient's discomfort, self extubation, removal of other lines and drains, or poor patient-ventilator synchrony. Too much sedation can also be harmful and can delay weaning.
- The RASS is a sedation agitation instrument that was developed to help titrate sedative medication and evaluate agitated behavior in the ICU patients.
- RASS will be completed on all intubated patients every four hours at a minimum. Inadequate sedation or over sedation should be reported promptly to the physician.
- RASS is a 10 point scale that ranges from +4 (combative) to -5 (unarousable). The score should be kept between -1 to -2. The values and definitions are:

  - +4 Combative
  - +3 Very agitated
  - +2 Agitated
  - +1 Restless
  - 0 Alert & calm
  - - 1 Drowsy
  - - 2 Light sedation
  - - 3 Moderate sedation
  - - 4 Deep Sedation
  - - 5 Unarousable

> **Note:** *it is important to discontinue all sedation every morning on the ventilated patient to reassess mental status and the need for continued sedation*

Safety

- Bag valve mask will be at the bedside for all ventilated patients.
- The head of the bed should be maintained at a 30-45 degree angle for all intubated patients unless contraindicated or otherwise ordered by physician.

Tracheostomy

- Trach care and inner cannula changes will be done every four hours and PRN for the first 48 hours with new tracheostomies. Routine trach care including inner cannula exchanges will occur once per shift and as needed.
- Obturator will remain at bedside and accompany patient if transported.

Chapter 19 **Respiratory drugs used in ventilator patients**

Pharmacological effects

These medications are most useful in patients with airway disease or airway infection. Effects include: bronchodilation (albuterol, ipratropium, levalbuterol); anti-inflammation (budesonide); antibiotic (tobramycin); mucolysis (N-acetylcysteine).

Delivery Systems

Special adapters (with T shape) are available to deliver nebulized (NEB) medication or metered dose inhaler (MDI) medication into the inspired gas limb of the ventilator circuit.

NEB

- Routine medications that can be nebulized can be given to a ventilated patient. The dosing is the same as that used routinely. Medications include:
  - Albuterol
  - Ipratropium
  - Levalbuterol (Xopenex)
  - Budesonide (only Pulmicort Respule)

MDI

- Only aerosol system MDI can be used; drugs in powder form such as Advair diskus cannot be used. The therapist must synchronize the medication delivery with the inhalation phase of the ventilator cycle for delivery. The use of MDI in ventilated patients is infrequent. Medications include:
  - ProAir (albuterol)
  - Combivent (albuterol/ipratropium)

Standard Dosing
Albuterol

- Dose: NEB: 2.5mg q3-6h. MDI: 2 puffs inhaled q4-6h
  Note: Patients who have severe bronchospasm and cannot be ventilated can be given albuterol more often or even continuously. However, they should be closely monitored. This should be prescribed by a specialist.

Ipratropium

- Dose: NEB 500 mcg q6-8h. MDI 2puffs inhaled q6h

Ipratropium/albuterol

- Dose: NEB: (DuoNeb) 500mcg/ 2.5mg q6h. MDI (Combivent) 1-2 puffs inhaled q6h

Budesonide
- Dose: NEB (Pulmicort Respules) 0.25mg or 0.5mg q12h
  Note: Not indicated to relieve acute bronchospasm. Dosing above 0.5mg per day may have some systemic steroid effects.

Levalbuterol.
- Dose: NEB 1.25 mg q6-8h. MDI 2 puffs inhaled q4-6h
  Note: it is an isomer of albuterol. It can be a useful alternative for patients with clinically significant side effects of albuterol such as tremor and tachycardia.

Tobramycin
- Dose: NEB: 300mg q12h for 30 days on and then 30 days off.
  Note: Usually reserved for Pseudomonas infections in patients with chronic airway diseases such as cystic fibrosis or bronchiectasis.

N-acetylcysteine
- Dose: NEB: 3-5 mL 20% sol or 6-10 mL 10% sol q6-8h
  Note: may be used to mobilize secretions. Give bronchodilator 10-15 min before the dose to avoid bronchospasm.

Goals for bronchodilator therapy
- ↓wheezing
- ↓secretions
- ↓peak pressure

Study Questions

How would you monitor the therapeutic effects of bronchodilators in a patient on a ventilator? Is there any rationale for using a beta-2 agonist in a patient on a ventilator with diffuse lung disease and no wheezes? Consider a patient on a ventilator with diffuse mucus plugging in the small airways. The patient is treated with N-acetylcysteine. What ventilator parameter might change if this medication had an important effect on the overall accumulation of secretion?

2001 American College of Critical Care Medicine (ACCM) **Sedation Guidelines** were developed to help guide the practitioner in the usage of sedatives and opiates for prolonged sedation and analgesia. Both sedation and analgesia should be administered to mechanically ventilated patients to achieve a level of comfort. The ACCM recommends the following drugs based on individual patient need.

Sedation

Lorazepam (Ativan)

- **Mechanism of action**-Binds to CNS GABA receptors and produces an inhibitory effect on neuronal excitability through hyperpolarization and stabilization.
- **Dose**-Start at 0.01-0.1 mg/kg/hr IV and titrate per RASS scale.
- **Pharmacokinetics** -Onset: IV 5 minutes. Metabolism: Hepatic to inactive compounds. Half-life elimination: Adults: 8-12 hours, prolonged with cirrhosis, congestive heart failure, obesity, usage > 72 hours, and elderly.
- **Pearls** - ACCM guidelines recommend lorazepam use for long term sedation (> 72 hr). Studies show that time to extubation was shorter with lorazepam than midazolam.

Midazolam (Versed)

- **Mechanism of action**- Binds to CNS GABA receptors and produces an inhibitory effect on neuronal excitability through hyperpolarization and stabilization.
- **Dose**-Start at 0.04-0.2 mg/kg/hour and titrate per RASS scale.
- **Pharmacokinetics**- Onset: IV 1-5 minutes. Metabolism: Extensively hepatic via CYP3A4 with active metabolite. Half-life elimination: 1-4 hours, prolonged with cirrhosis, congestive heart failure, obesity, usage > 72 hours, and elderly.
- **Pearls**-Good choice for short periods of sedation. Half-life of midazolam is profoundly increased when used > 72 hrs. Build-up of drug and active metabolite results in prolonged times to extubation once sedation is stopped.

Propofol (Diprivan)

- **Mechanism of action**- Propofol is a short-acting, lipophilic intravenous general anesthetic. Propofol causes global CNS depression, presumably through its agonist actions on $GABA_A$ receptors, and perhaps reduced glutamatergic activity through NMDA receptor blockade.
- **Dose**- 5 mcg/kg/minute; increase by 5-10 mcg/kg/min every 5-10 minutes until desired sedation level is achieved; usual maintenance dose of 10-40 mcg/kg/min.
- **Pharmacokinetics**- Onset: 30 seconds. Metabolism: Hepatic to water-soluble sulfate and glucuronide conjugates. Half-life elimination: Biphasic: Initial: 40 minutes; Terminal: 4-7 hours (after 10-day infusion, elimination may be up to 1-3 days).
- **Pearls**- Propofol is the drug of choice for short term sedation when rapid awakening is required. Always monitor triglyceride levels in patients receiving Propofol > 48hrs. Hypotension is common and rate limiting. Propofol usage > 72 hrs and at higher levels has resulted in Propofol infusion Syndrome (PIS) cases. PIS is marked by sudden bradycardia, progressing renal failure with rhabdomyolysis, and acute metabolic acidosis.

Dexmedetomidine (Precedex)

- **Mechanism of action** - Selective $alpha_2$-adrenoceptor agonist with anesthetic and sedative properties thought to be due to activation of G-proteins by $apha_{2a}$-adrenoceptors in the brainstem resulting in inhibition of norepinephrine.
- **Dose**-Initial: Loading infusion of 1 mcg/kg over 10 minutes followed by a maintenance infusion of 0.2-0.7 mcg/kg/hour; adjust rate to desired level of sedation; titration no more frequently than every 30 minutes may reduce the incidence of hypotension.
- **Pharmacokinetics**-Onset: 5-10 minutes. Duration: 60-120 minutes. Metabolism: Hepatic via N-glucuronidation, N-methylation, and CYP2A6.
- **Pearls**- Does not affect respiratory drive. Precedex is only FDA approved for 24 hour infusion duration. Hypotension occurs in 50% of patients and can be exacerbated by other anti-hypertensive medication. A difficult and expensive drug to use for sedation > 24 hours. Consider in patients who are difficult to wean secondary to agitation.

Comfort/Pain Control

Fentanyl

- **Mechanism of action** -Binds to opiate receptors in the CNS, causing inhibition of ascending pain pathways, altering the perception of and response to pain; produces generalized CNS depression.
- **Dose**-Continuous infusion: 50-700 mcg/hour or 0.7-10 mcg/kg/hour, Start opiate naive patients at 50-100 mcg/hr and titrate for pain/agitation control.
- **Pharmacokinetics** -Rapid onset- almost immediate. Duration: I.V.: 0.5-1 hour. Metabolism: Hepatic, primarily via CYP3A4. Half-life elimination: 2-4 hours.
- **Pearls**- Opiate of choice for rapid onset/discontinuation of analgesia, Opiate of choice for patients with hemodynamic instability and renal insufficiency.

Morphine

- **Mechanism of action** -Binds to opiate receptors in the CNS, causing inhibition of ascending pain pathways, altering the perception of and response to pain; produces generalized CNS depression.
- **Dose**- Continuous infusion: 5-35 mg/hour or 0.07-0.5 mg/kg/hour. Start opiate naive infusion at 5mg/hr and titrate for pain/agitation control.
- **Pharmacokinetics** -Onset of action: IV: 1-2 minutes. Metabolism: Hepatic via conjugation with glucuronic acid. Half-life elimination: 2-4 hours. Excretion: Metabolites in the urine.
- **Pearls**- Morphine is the preferred agent for intermittent therapy due to longer duration of action.

Add Notes or Questions

Chapter 21 **Common events and emergencies**

Common events with ventilated patients

- $\downarrow$ oxygen saturation
- Gurgling noise with every breath
- Low exhaled tidal volume alarm on ventilator
- $\uparrow$ plateau pressures
- $\uparrow$ peak pressures
- $\downarrow$ pressure or PEEP
- $\uparrow$ PCO_2/Respiratory acidosis
- Patient discomfort

Problems that need to be dealt with immediately (without waiting for CXR)

- Migration of ET tube (inwards or outwards)
- Blockage of ET tube
- Tension pneumothorax

Identifying a ventilator emergency

- **Clinical findings**
    - Dyspnea
    - Cyanosis
    - Diaphoresis
    - Absent or decreased breath sounds
- **May resolve if you**
    - Remove the patient from the ventilator
    - Bag manually with 100% O_2
    - Check ventilator connections and setting
    - Insert a catheter to the ETT to check for blockage

Outward migration of ET tube

- Physiology
    - Tidal volumes are not delivered
- Physical exam
    - ET tube marking at teeth usually significantly different
    - Cannot hear breath sounds when ventilating
    - Gurgling noise noted with each breath
- Ventilator findings
    - Expiratory tidal volume (V_{TE}) are very low or absent
    - High or low pressure alarm, depending on the position of tube
- Solution
    - Advance tube or replace tube
    - If you decide to advance the ET tube, do so only under direct vision with a laryngoscope or bronchoscope

Inward migration of ET tube
- Physiology
  - Results in right main stem intubation
  - Entire tidal volume goes to one lung and creates a shunt
- Physical exam
  - ET tube marking at teeth usually different
  - Asymmetric chest expansion/breath sounds. Usually more on right and less/absent on left
- Ventilator findings
  - May see high peak and plateau pressures
- Solution
  - Pull out tube (enough only, not all the way)

ET tube balloon rupture or failure
- Physiology
  - Tidal volume leaks around balloon, resulting in decreased tidal volumes and hypoventilation
- Physical exam
  - Gurgling sound with every breath
  - Decreased SaO_2
  - Inadequately inflated but properly functioning balloon, or an ETT with balloon above the vocal cords can present similarly
- Ventilator findings
  - Low exhaled tidal volume alarm on ventilator
- Solution
  - First try inflating the balloon. This usually solves the problem
  - Otherwise, need to replace ET tube

Other endotracheal tube related problems
- Patient biting on tube
  - Consider adjusting sedation
- Blocked tube from secretions/other causes
  - Frequent suctioning
- Failed connection
  - Adjust connection (by RT)

Non ETT related increase in airway resistance
- Sudden bronchospasm
  - Give bronchodilators
- Foreign bodies (very unlikely)
  - Remove foreign body

Tension Pneumothorax

- Physiology
    - Increased intrathoracic pressure impedes venous return, causing decreased or no cardiac output; impedes ventilation because of high pressure.
    - Result: anywhere from high pressures and decreased saturation to a frank cardiorespiratory arrest with electromechanical dissociation
- Physical exam
    - Unstable patient with no other explanation
    - Decreased saturation
    - Decreased breath sounds and resonant to percussion
    - Mediastinal shift to contralateral side: Trachea, PMI
    - Dilated neck veins
    - Difficult to "Bag"
- Ventilator findings
    - Increased peak and plateau pressures
    - Decreased exhaled tidal volumes
- Solution
    - Immediate needle/catheter decompression.
    - Second intercostals space: parasternal. Follow this with a tube thoracostomy.

Study Questions

List three reasons that patients might develop increased peak pressures.
List three reasons that patients might develop increased plateau pressures.
List three types of patients who might be at increased risk for tension pneumothorax.

Chapter 22 **Troubleshooting blood gases**

Low PaO$_2$ (O$_2$ saturation)

- ↑FiO$_2$ by 0.05-.10 increments
- ↑ PEEP by 2-3 cm H$_2$0
- ↑ I:E ratio by changing the inspiratory time (Ti)
- ↑Suctioning of secretions
- Use bronchodilators
- Use diuretics for pulmonary edema

High PaO$_2$ (O$_2$ saturation)

- ↓ FiO$_2$ in 0.05-.10 decrements

Acidosis/PaCO$_2$ increased

Secondary to ↓ $\dot{V}_E$ ($\dot{V}_E$ =V$_T$ x RR. Normal range is 5-8L/min)
- ↑V$_T$ by 1-2ml/kg IBW per hour (not higher than 10 ml/kg IBW)
- ↑ RR by 2-3 but do not exceed 35 breaths/min
- ↑ Peak pressure (on pressure support) to increase V$_T$ by 1-2 ml/kg IBW

Secondary to trauma, sepsis, burns, or high carbohydrates
- Correct underlying etiology
- Change diet to low carbohydrate, high fat

Alkalosis/PaCO$_2$ decreased

Secondary to ↑ $\dot{V}_E$
- ↓ RR by 2-3 breaths per minute
- ↓V$_T$ by 1-2ml/kg IBW
- ↓Peak pressure (on pressure support) by 5 cmH$_2$0

Secondary to ↑RR from anxiety, pain, CNS disorders
- ↑sedation
- ↑pain medication

Study Questions

A patient has been stable on the mechanical ventilation for six hours. A repeat ABG reveals a $PaCO_2$ of 60 mmHg and a pH 7.26. What are the potential explanations for this? How would you address this problem?

Chapter 23 **Troubleshooting pressure alarms**

↑ Peak pressure with normal plateau pressure

- Monitor will show a peak pressure **>40** cm H_2O and a plateau pressure **<30** cm H_2O
- Possible causes: ↑ secretions, bronchospasm, kinked tube
- Solution: suction, give bronchodilators, check tube

↑ Peak pressure with ↑ plateau pressure

- Monitor will show a peak pressure **>40** cm H_2O and a plateau pressure **>30** cm H_2O
- Possible causes: pneumothorax, ARDS, atelectasis, pulmonary edema, ETT in main bronchus
- Solution: treat the cause. Also try to ↓ pressures by ↓ V_T by 1-2 ml/kg IBW

↓ Plateau pressure

- Monitor will show a change in plateau pressure
- Possible causes: cuff leak, inadequate flow, disconnected tube, extubation
- Solution: inflate cuff, increase flow, check tubing, reintubate

$V_{TI} > V_{TE}$

- This indicates a leak
- For example, cuff not inflated enough or tracheoesophageal fistula
- Check cuff volume (pressure should be < 25 cm H_2O)
- If cuff is working, look for other causes

$MV_{IN} > MV_{EX}$

- Same concept as $V_{TI} > V_{TE}$

Case Analysis

Record the peak pressures and the plateau pressures on three separate patients while you are caring for them in the ICU. Look at trends over one day. Does this information provide any physiological conclusions about the patients' underlying lung diseases?

Chapter 24 **Weaning**

Consider weaning potential daily

- Patients intubated for a short period for surgery or drug OD generally do not need weaning
- Some patients can never be weaned. For example, advanced multiple sclerosis, ALS.
- Weaning trials should be tried only once per day. Studies have not demonstrated any benefit in trying to extubate a patient after several attempts during the same day.

Clinical indicators needed for possible weaning

- Hemodynamically stable
- Off all vasopressors
- $FiO_2 \leq 40\%$, PEEP ≤ 5
- Primary indication for mechanical ventilation improving
- Adequate Hb (≥ 10 g/dL), adequate K ≥ 3.5 mEq/L

Discontinue sedation

- Plan sedation management during the prior hospital day

Start spontaneous breathing trial (SBT)

- Usually CPAP (5cm H_2O) + pressure support (5 cm H_2O)
- Monitor clinical status, RR, HR, BP, sats for 30-120 minutes
- There is no benefit leaving a patient on a SBT longer than 120 minutes

Check weaning parameters at end of trial (bedside measurements by RT)

- RSBI (rapid shallow breathing index) $\leq$ **105** breaths/liter
  - Dividing the RR by the spontaneous V_{TE}
- Negative inspiratory force (NIF) more negative than - **20** cm H_2O
- Forced vital capacity (FVC) $\geq$ **10 ml/kg** IBW.

Check cuff leak (bedside measurements by RT)

- Helps identify patients at risk for post-extubation stridor who might require reintubation
- The difference between the V_{TI} and V_{TE} is checked with the ETT cuff deflated

- Greater than a 20% decrease in tidal volume indicates a leak
- Also checked by listening to the neck and hearing the leak
- No cuff leak may indicate laryngeal edema

If clinical status and numerical parameters are satisfactory, extubate

- Keep patient NPO for 8-24 hours
- Place on O_2 mask
- Encourage deep breaths and cough
- Monitor clinical status, RR, SaO_2, and voice quality

If clinical status and numerical parameters are NOT satisfactory, do not Extubate

- Resume sedation to keep the patient comfortable
- Resume original ventilator settings
- Monitor clinical status, RR, SaO_2
- Perform another weaning trial the following morning.

Study Question

Some patients on mechanical ventilators may require prolonged periods of time for weaning. What pathophysiological processes involving the lower respiratory tract or the respiratory muscles delay weaning? How might these various conditions be treated?

Chapter 25 Complications associated with mechanical ventilation

Immediate complications following intubation

- Hypoxia
- Hypotension
- Aspiration
- Injury to cervical spine

Airway complication/ ETT

- Direct injury to lips, tongue, teeth, pharynx, esophagus or trachea
- Tracheo-esophageal fistulas secondary to pressure necrosis by ETT in opposition to NGT.

GI complications

- Esophageal and gastric erosions or ulcers
- Constipation
- Abdominal distension

Physiologic changes with increased intrathoracic pressure

- Decreased cardiac output
- Decreased blood pressure
- Decreased urinary output
- Increased intracranial pressure

Ventilator-induced lung injury

- **Barotrauma-** over distention secondary to pressure
- **Volutrauma-** over distention secondary to volume

  Risk factors
    - Plateau >30 cmH$_2$O
    - Peak pressure >40 cmH$_2$O
    - V$_T$ > 12-15 ml/kg
    - PEEP >10-15 cmH$_2$O

Ventilator-associated pneumonia

- Refer to chapter 26

Oxygen toxicity

- It is not clear what concentration of inspired oxygen causes toxicity. The general principle is to reduce the FiO_2 to the lowest level that maintains a $PaO_2 > 55$ mmHg or $SaO_2 > 88\%$. Oxygen toxicity is associated with:

    ### Physiologic effects
    - Depression of respiratory drive
    - Pulmonary vasodilation
    - Ventilation-perfusion mismatch
    - Hypercarbia

    ### Pathological effects
    - Absorption atelectasis
    - Acute tracheobronchitis
    - Diffuse alveolar damage
    - ARDS
    - Bronchopulmonary dysplasia (in infants)

Post-extubation

- Throat pain
- Hoarseness
- Difficulty swallowing
- Withdrawal syndrome from opiates and benzodiazepines

Study Question

Consider the last three patients you managed on a mechanical ventilator. Did these patients have any complications during this care? Could these complications have been avoided?

Incidence

- Ventilator- associated pneumonias occur frequently (up to 70% after 30 days of mechanical ventilation). One older study demonstrated that the rate is approximately 1% per day of mechanical ventilation.

Definition

- These patients have a new or changing pulmonary infiltrate associated with purulent secretions, fever and leukocytosis. Most definitions require at least two of these three in addition to the infiltrate and no alternative diagnosis.

Microbiology

- If the patient has been on the ventilator for < 5 days the usual pathogens are the pathogens associated with community- acquired pneumonia. These would include *Streptococcus pneumonia*, *Haemophilus influenzae* and possibly atypical organisms such as Mycoplasma and Chlamydia.

- In patients on the ventilator for >5 days the usual pathogens are hospital-acquired pathogens, such as *Staphylococcus aureus*, Enterobactereacea spp (*E.coli*), *Pseudomonas aeruginosa*, and Acinetobacter spp. These organisms are frequently drug resistant.

Diagnosis

- Cultures can be obtained with tracheal suction specimens or bronchoalveolar lavage specimens using a non-directed "blind" catheter system or bronchoscopy with bronchoalveolar lavage or protected brush specimen. Most comparative studies indicate that outcomes using these methods to direct antibiotic therapy are similar.

Differential Diagnosis

- Atelectasis, pulmonary embolus, aspiration,
- pulmonary hemorrhage, atypical pulmonary edema

Treatment

- Broad spectrum coverage for Staphylococci and Gram-negative aerobic bacteria.
- Typical regimens would include three antibiotics

  - Vancomycin **or** linezolid **plus** extended-spectrum penicillin-beta lactam inhibitor combination **plus** an aminoglycoside **or** a fluoroquinolone.

  - Vancomycin **or** linezolid **plus** carbapenem **plus** an aminoglycoside **or** a fluoroquinolone.

  - Vancomycin **or** linezolid **plus** third **or** fourth generation cephalosporin **plus** an aminoglycoside **or** a fluoroquinolone.

- Broad spectrum coverage should be continued until culture results are available and then narrowed when possible to cover identified pathogens.

- Eight days of antibiotics is satisfactory if the patient has demonstrated improvement during the treatment course. Most Pseudomonas infections require 14 to 15 days of antibiotics.

Complications with ventilator-associated pneumonia

- Abscess formation
- Parapneumonic effusions

Outcomes

- Ventilator- associated pneumonias increase cost and length of stay. Treatment failure is high (25-40%). The attributable mortality is 25%.

Study Question

Your patient on a mechanical ventilator develops a new pulmonary infiltrate. What is the differential diagnosis? How would you evaluate this infiltrate?

Indications
Emergency tracheostomy
It is performed due to an anatomic obstacle preventing the establishment of a secure airway.

Planned tracheostomy
Prolonged endotracheal intubation can result in tracheal stenosis presumably due to ischemic injury of the trachea. Converting a patient from endotracheal intubation to tracheostomy should be considered if the patient has failed weaning on several attempts, if extubation trials have not been successful, or if the patient will require prolonged ventilator support. Benefits include easier access for tracheobronchial suctioning, patient comfort, lower or no sedation is needed, better patient communication, lower work of breathing, and management outside the ICU. The generally accepted standard is that patients should not have endotracheal tubes for longer than 14-21 days.

Procedure
Tracheostomy is performed by an ENT surgeon or general surgeon. The procedure may be performed in the operating room or at the bedside. One modern technique utilizes a fiberoptic scope to localize from inside the desired location. The surgeon then makes the external incision using the light source as the guide. Immediately after the tracheostomy is performed, the tube is vulnerable to being dislodged. Usually it is secured with ties to the skin. After about one week a tract will mature and the tube can be removed and re-inserted with minimal expertise. This permits training of the patient or family to care for the tracheostomy and clean the tube.

Cuff
Tracheostomy tubes can be divided into cuffed tubes and cuffless tubes. It is important to understand the pros and cons of both types. The cuff provides an air seal. This seal is necessary to inflate the respiratory system to high pressures. Controlled ventilation requires a cuff. Otherwise delivered volume is unreliable. The cuff is more prone to the formation of granulation tissue than the same size tube without a cuff. Cuffless tubes are easier to maintain and keep clean especially in the home setting. The other purpose for a cuff is to protect against aspiration. In general, cuffless tubes are appropriate only for patients who can sustain gas exchange on tracheostomy collar and who have passed swallow evaluations.

Fenestrated Tubes

Fenestrations are placed to permit airflow out of the tracheostomy tube and through the vocal cords to permit speech. Fenestrations may be used with speaking valves to maintain ventilation most of the time when speech is not desired. The main challenges with fenestrations are that tube position becomes more critical to function and the fenestration is prone to being clogged by granulation tissue.

Tracheostomy Buttons

Some patients do not need a tracheostomy at the current moment but are at very high risk for needing airway access in the future. These patients may use a button to maintain the tracheostomy stoma and tract in between periods of tracheostomy use. The tracheostomy stoma and tract will close in a matter of a few days unless it is kept open by a physical device.

Ventilation and Tracheostomy Tubes

Cuffed tubes are ventilated in the same manner as endotracheal tubes. In general cuffless tubes require the patient to ventilate himself as positive pressure ventilation will leak around the tube. Negative pressure ventilation with an iron lung or a cuirass can be done with a cuffless tube. Limited ventilator assistance can be given as pressure support with a relatively tight fitting cuffless tube. Some ventilators, similar to devices used for CPAP, require a controlled leak to function properly and these are suitable for limited ventilator assistance with cuffless tubes.

Tracheostomy Weaning

Once the patient can protect his airway and can sustain gas exchange without ventilator assistance, the patient can be weaned from the tracheostomy tube. The usual criteria would be satisfactory performance on tracheostomy collar and swallow testing. The tracheostomy tube should be downsized to a smaller caliber cuffless tube. This will permit easy flow of air around the tube through the vocal cords. The performance of the upper airway is tested by capping the tracheostomy tube. If the patient can ventilate and oxygenate without distress while the tracheostomy tube is capped, the tube can be removed and the stoma and tract can be allowed to heal.

Study question

Deciding when to do a tracheostomy in a patient requiring mechanical ventilation can be a complex decision. Can you provide any general principle for this decision?

Dysphagia
Etiologies
- Injury from intubation, cricothyrotomy, tracheostomy
- Post-extubation glottic edema, laryngospasm
- Prolonged pharmacologic effects of sedatives and muscle relaxants
- Up to 50% of elderly patients ($\geq$65) have an abnormal swallow after orotracheal intubation for more than 48 hours

Diagnosis
- Barium swallow with video fluoroscopy
- Esophageal manometry
- Endoscopy

Treatment
- Diet alteration, speech therapy
- Temporary gastrostomy

Tracheal Stenosis
Epidemiology
- Documented evidence of positive tomogram in 19% of patients with endotracheal intubation and 65% patients with tracheostomy
- Advanced, asymptomatic stenosis (25% decrease in diameter) seen in first few months of 25-40% patients after decannulation
- Increased cuff pressure with mucosal injury occurs within 15 minutes when lateral wall pressures rise beyond 27 cm H_2O

Diagnosis
- Stridor, wheeze, decreased lung sounds, inadequate or increased work for breathing
- Symptoms occur when lumen is decreased by >30% of its original diameter. Dyspnea can develop when the lumen becomes 10 mm in diameter and stridor when the diameter is 5mm or less.
- Imaging: laryngeal tomogram, chest CT
- Bronchoscopy for direct visualization

Treatment
- Prevention by monitoring cuff pressures to keep below 30 cm H_2O
- Mild stenosis can be treated conservatively with oxygen, respiratory therapy, and antibiotics in case of infection

- Endoscopic options
  - Tracheal dilation
  - Transluminal stent placement
  - Laser ablation
- Open tracheal reconstruction using stents (autologous, homologous, or inert)

Delirium
Epidemiology
- Prevalence in post extubated patients is unknown
- Types of delirium: 2% hyperactive, 44% hypoactive, 54% for mixed
- Number of days of delirium positively correlates with longer duration of mechanical ventilation, prolonged neurophysiological dysfunction, and increased post hospital mortality

Pathophysiology/Risk Factors
- Theorized underlying mechanisms:
  - Imbalance of neurotransmitters
  - Inflammatory mediators
  - Impaired oxidative metabolism
  - Cholinergic deficiency (impaired Ach production secondary to hypoxia)
  - Dysfunction of central sodium-dependent neuronal amino acid transporters
- Risk factors: advanced age, comorbid conditions, baseline cognitive impairment, genetic predisposition, hypoxia, sepsis, metabolic disturbances, anticholinergic medications, sedatives, sleep disturbances

Diagnosis
- CAM-ICU (Confusion Assessment Method for the ICU): monitor mental status
- ICU Memory Tool: eight question survey to evaluate recall of factual and delusional memories

Treatment
- Improve patient orientation with cognitive therapy
- Normalizing sleep/wake cycles
- Early mobilization
- Correct underlying problem (e.g., hypoxia, hypercarbia, etc.)
- Benzodiazepines are not recommended
- Anecdotal evidence supports use of haloperidol as cited by Society of Critical Care

Posttraumatic Stress Disorder
Definition
- Constellation of symptoms in three domains
  - Reexperiencing
  - Avoidance/emotional numbing
  - Increased arousal

Epidemiology
- Prevalence varies widely 5-64% and often misdiagnosed
- Delayed onset of PSTD symptoms in 16% of discharged ICU patients
- Prevalence higher in certain subpopulations (e.g., ARDS) ranging from 25 to 40%

Pathophysiology/Risk Factors
- Risk factors: delusional ICU memories, a greater number of traumatic memories, extended ICU stay, longer duration of mechanical ventilation, younger age, prior mental health history, female gender, higher levels of sedation and neuromuscular blockade
- Development of symptoms is multifactorial: profound feelings of helplessness during time of illness, pre-existing psychiatric condition, cognitive impairment with decreased working memory, and multiple traumatic events (pain, panic, respiratory distress, nightmares)

Diagnosis
- PTSS-14 (Post Traumatic Stress Syndrome 14 questionnaire)
- IES-R (Impact of Events Scale-Revised): evaluates stress reaction from prolonged ICU hospitalization

Treatment
- Absence of episodic memory for a traumatic event is protective against the development of PTSD
- Cognitive behavioral therapy considered first line treatment and has long-term efficacy

Depression
Epidemiology
- Incidence is unknown in post-extubated patients

Diagnosis
- Criteria to meet: one of two core symptoms of depressed mood or reduced interest plus five of the following:
  - Insomnia or hypersomnia, reduced interest/pleasure, excessive guilt/feelings of worthlessness, reduced energy, decreased concentration, loss of either appetite or weight, psychomotor agitation, and suicidal behavior
- Survey instruments:
  - GDS-SF (Geriatric Depression Scale-Short Form)
  - BDI (Beck Depression Inventory)
  - CES-D (Center for Epidemiologic Studies Depression Scale)
  - HADS (Hospital Anxiety-Depression Scale)

Treatment
- Pharmacologic: TCA, SSRI, SNRI, or NRI
- Psychiatry referral

Anxiety
Epidemiology
- 23–48% of ALI/ARDS survivors have clinically significant nonspecific anxiety symptoms

Risk Factors
- Advanced age
- Female gender
- Length of ICU stay

Diagnosis
- HADS (Hospital Anxiety-Depression Scale)
- BAI (Beck Anxiety Inventory)

Treatment
- Correct underlying problem (e.g., hypoxemia, hypotension, hypoglycemia)
- Analgesics, SSRI, SNRI, benzodiazepines

Profound Muscle Weakness
Definition
- Neuromuscular degeneration during ICU care resulting in weakness and/or paralysis
- May delay weaning and rehabilitation
- Critical illness polyneuropathy often considered a manifestation of multiple organ failure

Epidemiology
- Two-thirds of ARDS patients experience muscular weakness
- 25-30% incidence in patients requiring mechanical ventilation for more than 4 days
- 50-60% patients recover completely within 6 months

Pathophysiology
- Release of cytokine and low-molecular-weight neurotoxins during sepsis leads to axonal degeneration and probable insult to myelin
- Alternatively, isolated myopathy may develop in patients being treated with corticosteroids or neuromuscular blocking agents (possibly due to up-regulation of receptors after medical denervation with paralytic agents)
- Electrolyte disturbances: hypophosphatemia, hypomagnesemia, hypercalcemia

Diagnosis
- Muscle wasting
- Loss of deep tendon reflexes, temperature, pressure and vibration sensation
- Electromyography: detection of denervation changes (most marked in distal muscles) such as fibrillation potentials, positive sharp waves, and reduced motor unit recruitment
- Biopsy is the gold standard

Treatment
- There are no proven therapies but studies have suggested the following:
  - Remove offending agent
  - Treat underlying problem
  - Adequate nutrition
  - Supportive care with clinical follow up and physical therapy

Malnutrition

Epidemiology
- Most patients have inadequate oral intake for the first 7 days after extubation

Treatment
- Periodic calorie intake review
- Dietary consultation

Study Question

Most patients who require mechanical ventilation with endotracheal intubation have dysphagia and reduced caloric intake following extubation. Outline the strategies which help manage these problems.

Chapter 29 **Annotated bibliography of selected studies by the ARDS Network**

The ARDS Network is a clinical research network of approximately 42 hospitals, organized into twelve clinical sites, and a coordinating center. The Principal Investigators from each site together with the NHLBI Project Scientists form the Network Steering Committee, the main governing body of the Network. The Steering Committee is responsible for identification of promising new agents for the treatment of ARDS, setting Network priorities, developing protocols, facilitating the conduct and monitoring of the trials, and reporting study results. A Protocol Review Committee provides an independent scientific evaluation for the NHLBI on each new protocol. The Data and Safety Monitoring Board monitors the conduct of the trial and advises the NHLBI on the quality of the trial and may suggest early termination of the study for either unanticipated large beneficial effects or for safety concerns. (Copied from the ARDS network website-ardsnet.org- accessed 1/5/2011)

1. The Acute Respiratory Distress Syndrome Network. Ventilation with **lower tidal volumes** as compared with traditional tidal volumes for acute lung injury and the acute respiratory distress syndrome. N Engl J Med 2000; 342: 1301-1308.
    This pivotal study reported the outcome in 861 patients in a randomized controlled trial which compared a low tidal volume strategy (6ml/kg IBW) with a plateau pressure < 30 cm H_2O against a conventional tidal volume strategy (12ml/kg IBW) with a plateau pressure <50 cm H_2O. The absolute mortality difference was 8.8% (NNT= 11). This now represents the standard of care in ARDS.

2. Brower RG, et al. **Higher versus lower positive end-expiratory pressures** in patients with the acute respiratory distress syndrome. N Engl J Med 2001; 351: 327-36.

This study randomized 549 patients with acute lung injury into either a high PEEP (13 cm H_2O) or a low PEEP (8 cm H_2O) protocol. All patients were ventilated with a low tidal volume (6 ml/Kg IBW)) and a controlled plateau pressure (<30 cm H_2O) strategy. There was no difference in mortality.

3. Brower RG, et al. Effects of **recruitment maneuvers** in patients with acute lung injury and acute respiratory distress syndrome ventilated with high positive end-expiratory pressure. Crit Care Med. 2004 Mar;32(3):907.

72 patients with acute lung injury underwent either active recruitment maneuvers (CPAP 35-40 cmH_2O for 30 seconds) or sham recruitment maneuvers. The mean increase in SpO_2 was 1.7 % at 10 minutes post maneuver. This increase did not persist, and there were no long term benefits. This maneuver did not cause barotrauma.

4. Hager DN, et al. Tidal volume reduction in patients with acute lung injury when **plateau pressures are not high**. Am J Respir Crit Care Med 2005; 172: 1241-5.

This analysis suggests that there is no "safe" upper limit of plateau pressure. However, reducing the tidal volume when the plateau pressure is already low may not be warranted as hypercapnea has physiological consequences.

5. Eisner MD, et al. Airway pressures and **early barotrauma** in patients with acute lung injury and acute respiratory distress syndrome. Am J Respir Crit Care Med 2001; 165: 978-82.

This study retrospectively examined the risk factors for early barotrauma in 718 ARDS/ALI patients. The cumulative incidence of barotrauma was 13 % during the first four days of ventilation. Higher concurrent PEEP was associated with an increased risk of barotrauma with a relative hazard of 1.67 per 5 cm H_2O increase in PEEP.

6. Steinberg KP, et al. Efficacy and safety of **corticosteroids** for persistent acute respiratory distress syndrome. N Engl J Med 2006; 354: 1671-84. **180 patients with ARDS for at least seven days received either methylprednisolone or placebo. The methylprednisolone regimen included a loading dose, 0.5 mg per kg every 6 hours for 14 days, and then a taper. Methylprednisolone improved oxygenation, respiratory system compliance, and blood pressure but did not improve mortality at 60 days. If started after 14 days of ARDS, it increased mortality. This study does not support the routine use of methylprednisolone.**

7. Wiedemann HP, et al. Comparison of two **fluid-management** strategies in acute lung injury. N Engl J Med 2006; 354: 2564-75. **This randomized trial compared the outcomes with either a conservative or a liberal fluid strategy in 1,000 patients with acute lung injury. The protocol was complex and resulted in a fluid balance at 7 days of -136 ml in the conservative fluid arm and + 6992 ml in the liberal arm group. There was no difference in mortality at 60 days. A conservative strategy did not increase the frequency of shock or the use of dialysis but did increase oxygenation and reduce the lung injury score.**

8. Wheeler AP, et al. **Pulmonary-artery versus central venous catheter** to guide treatment of acute lung injury. N Engl J Med 2006; 354: 2213-24.

   1000 patients were randomized into hemodynamic management protocols using either a pulmonary artery catheter or a central venous catheter. There were no differences in fluid balance, hypotension, use of vasopressors or dialysis, or mortality at 60 days. Patients with pulmonary artery catheters had more complications.

9. Rice TW, et al. Comparison of the **SpO_2/FIO_2 ratio** and the PaO2/FIO2 ratio in patients with acute lung injury or ARDS. Chest 132:410-417, 2007.

   This study reports a secondary analysis of 2613 measurements of oxygen saturation, PaO_2 and FiO_2. The equation for the relationship between the SpO_2/FiO_2 and PaO_2/FiO_2 was: $SpO_2/FiO_2 = 64 + 0.84 \times PaO_2/FiO_2$ (r=0.89). If $SpO_2/FiO_2 = 235$, then $PaO_2/FiO_2 = 200$; if $SpO_2/FiO_2 = 315$, then $PaO_2/FiO_2 = 300$. Therefore, the SpO_2/FiO_2 ratio is a reliable indicator of PaO_2/FiO_2.

10. Cooke CR, et al. A simple clinical predictive index for objective estimates of **mortality** in acute lung injury. Crit Care Med 2009; 1913-20.

    This study reports a secondary analysis of simple variables in 873 patients to develop a model to predict mortality. The variable in model were: age <39 yrs-0 points, 40-64yrs-1 pt, >65 yrs-2 pts; bilirubin > 2mg/dl-1 pt; Hct< 26%-1 pt; fluid balance in 24 hr >2500 ml-1 pt. The mortality predictions were: 0 pts-8%, 1 pt-17%, 2 pts-31%, 3 pts-51 %, 4-5 pts-70%.

Chapter 30 **Short case reviews**

1. Indications for mechanical ventilation

A 32 year otherwise healthy female is admitted for dysuria and fever. She is admitted to the floor for IV antibiotics. A critical care consult is requested at 1AM because of low blood pressure. The resident orders a 3000 ml of NS in addition to appropriate antibiotics. The patient continues to be hypotensive despite the fluids and vasopressors, and is transferred to the ICU. She now complains of respiratory distress. She is still hypotensive and is in obvious significant distress. ABG shows a pH 7.45, pCO_2 35, HCO_3 22 and SaO_2 of 95% on 40% FiO_2. CXR shows bilateral infiltrates. Regarding her respiratory status, the next appropriate step is to:

- A. Place her on 100% NRB
- B. Obtain another ABG and CXR in 30-60 minutes to decide further course of action. Intubate if she shows significant hypoxemia or abnormal CXR.
- C. Intubate and initiate mechanical ventilation immediately
- D. Obtain another ABG and CXR in 30-60 minutes to decide further course of action. Intubate if she shows significant respiratory acidosis or abnormal CXR.

2. Initial Setup: Modes

A decision is made to intubate and place the above patient on mechanical ventilation. Which of the following ventilation modes would be your initial choice?

- A. Assist Control
- B. Synchronized Intermittent Mechanical Ventilation
- C. Airway Pressure Release Ventilation
- D. Pressure Control Ventilation (CPAP)
- E. High Frequency Oscillatory Ventilation

3. Initial Setup: Settings

She weighs 100 kg and is 5'6" tall. The recommended tidal volume for her is:

- A. 1000 ml
- B. 750 ml
- C. 600 ml
- D. 360 ml
- E. None of the above.

4. The initial PEEP, FiO_2 and RR settings for her could be:

- A. PEEP 0, FiO_2 40%, RR 12
- B. PEEP 5, FiO_2 20%, RR 18
- C. PEEP 15, FiO_2 100%, RR 36
- D. PEEP 5, FiO_2 100%, RR 24

87

5. Ventilator Settings: Adjustments

The patient above is placed on a V_T of 360, RR of 20, PEEP of 12 and FiO_2 of 100%. Her SaO_2 now is 72%. What do you do next?

A. Increase FiO_2
B. Increase PEEP
C. Change to APRV
D. Change to PRVC
E. Increase Tidal Volumes

6. Ventilator Settings: Adjustments

Appropriate changes in PEEP are made. SaO_2 has now come up to 78% and the patient appears uncomfortable. What do you do next?

A. Increase PEEP further
B. Sedate patient
C. Increase FiO_2
D. Change mode to APRV

7. Ventilator Settings: Adjustments

Appropriate action is taken. Two hours later, her BP is 110/75, HR 98, RR 30/minute, her plateau pressure is 29, her peak airway pressure is 35, SaO_2 is 94% but the ABGs show a pH of 7.25 with a pure respiratory acidosis. The next step is to:

A. Increase tidal volume
B. Decrease tidal volume
C. Decrease rate
D. Start an IV bicarbonate infusion to maintain a pH 7.35-7.45
E. Do nothing at this point

8. Ventilators: Troubleshooting

Appropriate steps are taken. Later in the day the nurse calls you because of high pressure alarms on the ventilator and decreased SaO_2. You notice an obviously awake patient in distress. The immediate next steps will include all ***except:***

A. Order a stat CXR and wait for the CXR before taking the next step
B. Remove patient from the ventilator and "manually bag the patient"
C. Sedate the patient to prevent asynchronous breathing and straining
D. Note the ease or difficulty in "bagging" the patient
E. Auscultate and percuss for symmetry
F. Note position of ET tube to look for migration

9. Ventilators: Troubleshooting

A 68 year male who was admitted for pneumonia is currently on mechanical ventilation (AC, V_T 360, RR 12, PEEP 5, FiO_2 55%). Patient is breathing at 26/minute. You are concerned about the significant respiratory alkalosis that this patient has. You will address this by making the following change:

A. Increase FiO_2 to decrease the respiratory drive
B. Decrease respiratory rate
C. Decrease PEEP
D. Increase sensitivity for triggering the ventilator
E. None of the above

10. Ventilator: Modes

A 55 year male with advanced COPD presents with respiratory distress, cough, and fever. Physical examination shows a mild fever, bilateral wheezing, and respiratory distress. ABGs show pO_2 50, pH 7.25, pCO_2 60. He is awake and able to follow commands. Steroids and bronchodilators are started. It is appropriate to place the patient on:

A. Oxygen alone
B. Noninvasive mechanical ventilation
C. Invasive mechanical ventilation

11. Ventilators: Discontinuing

During weaning, a patient is found to have a V_T of 400 cc and a RR of 20. The RSBI (Rapid Shallow Breathing Index) for this patient is:

A. 20
B. 8000
C. 50
D. Cannot be calculated based on the information available

12. Ventilation: Discontinuing

A 67 year female is admitted to the ICU for urosepsis and ARDS. On the fifth ICU day she is afebrile and appears awake and comfortable. She is on Zosyn, vancomycin, Lovenox, Nexium, dopamine (15mcg/kg/min), versed and Fentanyl. She is on AC, V_T 360cc, PEEP 5, FiO_2 35%, RR 16/min. Weaning parameters show a NIF of -65 and RSBI of 45.

A. Extubate patient
B. Do not extubate patient

13. Ventilation: Discontinuing

A 75 year old male is admitted with pneumonia and ARDS. On the sixth admission day, he is afebrile and appears awake and comfortable. He is on Zosyn, vancomycin, Lovenox, Nexium, Versed and Fentanyl. He is on AC, V_T 340ml, FiO_2 75%, RR 16/min, PEEP 12.5. Weaning parameters show a NIF of -75 and a RSBI of 44.

    A.   Extubate patient
    B.   Do not extubate patient

14. Ventilator: Discontinuing

A 34 year male with progressive GBS (bulbar) is intubated because of inability to protect airway and severe respiratory acidosis. Ten days later, his neurological condition has not deteriorated further and is unchanged otherwise. He is afebrile, awake and looks quite comfortable. He is hemodynamically stable, has a clear CXR, and has very good oxygenation.

    A.   Extubate patient
    B.   Do not extubate patient

15. Ventilator: Discontinuing

A 45 year male with aspiration pneumonia is admitted for respiratory failure. He is intubated and placed on mechanical ventilation. 7 days later, he is hemodynamically stable, off vasopressors, and has a SaO_2 of 94% on a FiO_2 of 35%. He tolerates PSV, PS 5cm and PEEP 5cm for 2 hours. Weaning parameters show a NIF of -55, V_T of 200 ml and RR of 40.

    A.   Extubate patient
    B.   Do not extubate patient

16. Ventilator: Discontinuing

A 45 year male with cirrhosis is admitted for alcohol withdrawal and is intubated for airway protection. Three days later, he is no longer agitated. He is hemodynamically stable and the labs are all within normal limits. The Ativan drip that patient was on has been discontinued and he is unarousable. His SaO_2 is 99%. He is on AC, V_T 400 ml, RR 18/min, FiO_2 25%, PEEP 5. Weaning parameters show a RSBI of 35.

    A.   Extubate patient
    B.   Do not extubate patient

1. **Answer: C**

Rationale:

While significant hypoxia and hypercarbia that does not respond to other conservative measures are reasonable indications for initiating mechanical ventilation, these are not the only one. It is reasonable to control the airway and initiate mechanical ventilation even in the absence of significant hypoxia in the following circumstances: (1) Significant and severe respiratory distress. Most of these patients will eventually develop frank respiratory failure if no intervention is carried out early (2) Significant hemodynamic instability that is likely to get worse. Severe hypotension will eventually affect mentation, control of airway, and respiratory effort.

The patient in question has septic shock and is developing ARDS. She is hypotensive despite reasonable doses of vasopressors, and has respiratory distress. Cardiorespiratory arrest is likely if her airway and ventilation are not controlled.

If you cannot remember any other indications, remember: If you are not sure and your patient looks "really bad," go ahead and intubate and ventilate, irrespective of ABGs. In such a situation, the technical description for the "indication for intubation" would be "For control of airway, and because of impending cardiorespiratory collapse."

2. **Answer: A**

Rationale:

AC is the most appropriate mode for initiating ventilation for practically all patients. SIMV offers no benefit in terms of initial mode of ventilation, and has the potential for inducing patient discomfort if all breaths are not supported. PSV/CPAP is not appropriate because this patient will likely lose her respiratory drive and hence her ability to initiate ventilation very soon and will have worsening lung compliance, translating in progressively decreasing tidal volumes at a given PS setting. APRV could be a consideration but is more complicated and provides no additional benefit. This patient does not meet criteria for HFOV as yet.

AC can be used for practically all circumstances, except as a weaning mode.

3. **Answer: D**
4. **Answer: D**

Rationale:

PEEP: Most patients have hypoxia, and so a non-zero relatively low PEEP as the initial setting is probably appropriate. 5 as the initial setting is probably reasonable. This can be adjusted up later. Higher initial settings of PEEP are acceptable for ARDS patients or those significantly hypoxic.

FiO$_2$: It is reasonable to start at a FiO$_2$ at 100% and titrate down based on patient requirements.

Resp Rate: A rate comparable to what the patient was breathing before intubation, but not very high is reasonable. 18-24 as the initial setting is reasonable.

Tidal Volume: ARDS patients benefit from a low tidal volume in terms of survival. 6 ml/Kg of IDEAL and not ACTUAL body weight is recommended. You may go as high as 8ml/Kg, but 6 ml/Kg is probably more appropriate. Tidal volumes can be higher for non ARDS like conditions where the lungs are not stiff, such as depressed sensorium and neuromuscular processes. No controlled studies exist for obstructive airway disorders, but smaller tidal volumes are better than larger tidal volumes because of the potential for dynamic hyperinflation. Therefore, while the 6ml/Kg V$_T$ for IDEAL body weight comes from ARDS data, this number is probably appropriate for severe obstructive airway disorders as well.

5. **Answer: B**

Rationale:

A very common reason for patients to continue to be hypoxic is because they do not have adequate PEEP. The table below from the ARDS net trials provides acceptable PEEP and FiO$_2$ combinations. PEEP should be raised as the FiO$_2$ requirements go up. While the tables go all the way up to 24, if you have to use more than 15 cm of PEEP, talk to someone who is more familiar with ventilators. (0.5=50%)

ARDS Net original PEEP/ FiO$_2$ combination recommendation

SaO$_2$ (%)	80	82	84	86	88	90	92	93	94	95	96	97	98	99
PaO$_2$(mmHg)	44	46	49	52	55	60	65	69	73	79	86	96	112	145

6. **Answer: B**

Rationale:
Patient discomfort and agitation causes "Patient Ventilator Dys-synchrony," reducing the effective ventilation. Appropriate sedation improves ventilation in these patients. Paralysis may be required briefly early on for some of these patients.

7. **Answer: E**

Rationale:

The concept of "permissive hypercapnia" is important to recognize. Except for patients who have an increased intracranial pressure, pregnant patients and those with unstable arrhythmias or severe hemodynamic instability, most patients tolerate a relatively high PCO_2 and a relatively low pH quite well. In fact, permissive hypercapnia would be preferable in patients who do not have the contraindications above, and are hard to ventilate because the risks of baro/volu trauma in these patients far outweigh the benefits, if any, of normalizing the pH and PCO_2. It is not clear as to what the target pH should be in these patients. Most of these patients tolerate a pH as low as 7.2 or 7.25 quite well. pH is probably a better parameter to watch than the pCO_2.

8. Answer: A
Rationale:
Refer to the section titled "troubleshooting". Bottom line, don't wait for CXR to rule out tube malposition or tension pneumothorax. Your patient may be dead by the time you get the CXR.

9. Answer: E
Rationale:
Every time a patient is on AC and triggers the ventilator, the ventilator delivers the full tidal volume. So if the patient is over-breathing the ventilator, decreasing the backup/set rate will have no impact on the final respiratory rate and the minute ventilation. The two ways to decrease the minute ventilation would be either to decrease the sensitivity so that the patient cannot trigger the ventilator, or to decrease the respiratory drive of the patient by sedating her/him. Decreasing sensitivity of ventilator triggering will work but is uncomfortable. So sedation is the way to go for this patient.

10. Answer: B
Rationale:
This patient needs mechanical ventilation because of respiratory failure. Non-invasive ventilation would be the ventilation of choice because it reduces mortality, ICU stay and the need for invasive ventilation in these patients as long as the patient is awake and cooperative, the mask can be placed on the face/nose, and the patient can be monitored closely for clinical improvement/deterioration. These patients should be in the ICU and should be re-evaluated in no more than 30-60 minutes later to decide if invasive ventilation is needed.

"BIPAP" is the ventilation mode to use. This is actually a PSV (Pressure Support Ventilation) with PEEP. So if you place the patient on "BIPAP 10/5", in essence, the patient is on a PEEP of 5 and Pressure Support of 5. The PEEP improves oxygenation and the PS drives tidal volumes. BIPAP 10/5 or 12/6 are reasonable initial settings.

11. Answer: C

Rationale:

RSBI is the ratio of the RR and V_T (in liters). So here, the RSBI is 20/0.4 = 50. RSBI is low when the patient is breathing slowly and has high tidal volumes. It is high when patient is "panting." RSBI less than 100 predicts a greater likelihood of success than when the RSBI is high. RSBI is not the only criterion that should be used to assess eligibility for extubation.

Other weaning parameters include

1. Negative Inspiratory Force (NIF) of better (more negative) than -20,
2. Forced Vital Capacity > 10 mg/Kg Ideal body weight,
3. Spontaneous minute volume < 10 l/min,
4. Spontaneous respiratory rate < 25/minute and
5. Spontaneous V_T of > 5 ml/Kg IBW.

12. Answer: B

Rationale:

Patients with hemodynamic should not be extubated. Ongoing need for vasopressors in this patient disqualifies her for extubation.

13. Answer: B

Rationale:

Patients should have acceptable oxygenation and reasonable low PEEP and FiO_2 requirements before extubation. This patient needs too high a PEEP and FiO_2 to be extubated successfully. Patients needing a PEEP of > 5 and a FiO_2 of more than 40% should in general not be extubated.

14. Answer: B

Rationale:

The underlying condition that formed the basis for intubation/ventilation for this patient should have reversed for you to consider extubation. This is not so in this patient.

15. Answer: B

Rationale:

RSBI is too high for this extubation to be successful.

16. Answer: B

Rationale:

Patients need to be awake, responsive, and able to protect the airway and clear secretions for the extubation to be successful. This patient does not meet those criteria.

Chapter 32 **Glossary**

1. **ALI:** acute lung injury, PaO_2/FiO_2 <300

2. **Airflow Resistance (R_{aw}):** a major factor that determines the rates of airflow in the airways. R_{aw} is equal to the sum of the resistance of all airways from the trachea to the alveolus. It is increased with bronchospasm or secretions.

3. **ARDS:** acute respiratory distress syndrome, PaO_2/FiO_2 <200

4. **CMV:** controlled mandatory ventilation. Every breath is mandatory.

5. **Dual control:** two variables are control by independent feedback loops.

6. **FiO_2:** fraction of inspired oxygen in a gas mixture. It is expressed as a number from 0=0% to 1=100%. FiO_2 on room air is 0.21=21%; pure oxygen is 1.0 = 100%.

7. **Flow rate:** inspiratory flow delivered by the ventilator during inspiration. 60mL/min is usually enough.

8. **I:E ratio:** the ratio of inspiratory time to expiratory time. Normally maintained at 1:2-3. This will allow the patient to passively exhale the large volumes employed during mechanical ventilation.

9. **IMV:** intermittent mandatory ventilation. Machine–triggered breaths with spontaneous breaths allowed in between.

10. **Lung Compliance (C_L)** is a measure of the elastic properties of the lung. It measures how easily the lung distends. High lung compliance is a lung that distends easily, and low lung compliance is a "stiff" lung.

11. **MAP:** mean airway pressure is the average pressure to which the lungs are exposed to during the respiratory cycle. It reflects mean alveolar pressure. It is associated with alveolar ventilation, arterial oxygenation, hemodynamic performance, and barotrauma.

12. **Minute ventilation ($\dot{V}_E$).** $\dot{V}_E = V_T \times RR$

13. **$PaCO_2$** (partial pressure of carbon dioxide) reflects the amount of carbon dioxide gas dissolved in the plasma. Normal range 35-45 mmHg.

14. **PaO$_2$** (partial pressure of arterial oxygen) reflects pressure exerted by free oxygen molecules dissolved in plasma. It reflects the efficiency of gas exchange.

15. **PAO$_2$** (partial pressure of alveolar oxygen) reflects the partial pressure of oxygen in the alveolar space.

16. **(PAO$_2$ - PaO$_2$) gradient.** It is the difference between measured PaO$_2$ and calculated PAO$_2$. It is used as an indirect measure of ventilation-perfusion abnormalities. Formula: PAO$_2$-PaO$_2$. PaO$_2$ from the ABG; PAO$_2$ = (760-47) x FiO$_2$ – PaCO$_2$/0.8 Normal : room air 5-20 mmHg; 100%FiO$_2$ 25-65 mmHg

17. **PaO$_2$/PAO$_2$ ratio** is the same information as above but expressed as a ratio. Normal range: 0.75-0.95.

18. **PaO$_2$ / FiO$_2$** is a ratio used to define acute lung injury and ARDS. At sea level it is normal range is 350-450 mmHg. In acute lung injury <300 mmHg, in ARDS <200mmHg.

19. **Peak pressure:** maximum pressure during the inspiratory phase of the cycle.

20. **PEEP**: positive end-expiratory pressure.

21. **pH** it is a measurement used to designate the acid-base balance of the blood and reflects the number of hydrogen ions present. Normal range is 7.35-7.45.

22. **PiO$_2$**: Inspired partial pressure of oxygen. PiO2=FiO$_2$ (Patm – 47 mm Hg). Where Patm is the atmospheric pressure (760 mmHg at sea level).

23. **Plateau pressure**: is the pressure at the end of inspiration during a period of no airflow.

24. **Pressure control:** the ventilator maintains a preset airway pressure throughout inspiration.

25. **PSV:** pressure support ventilation. Every breath is spontaneous and supported to a preset inspiratory pressure.

26. *RASS:* Richmond agitation sedation scale is a monitoring tool that is used to help titrate sedation appropriately in the ICU.

27. **RSBI:** Rapid Shallow Breathing Index is calculated by dividing the respiratory rate by the spontaneous expiratory tidal volume (V_{TE}). It is expressed in liters, e.g.,30/0.3 = 100.

28. **SBT**: Spontaneous Breathing Trial.

29. **SIMV**: synchronized intermittent mandatory ventilation. Patient or machine triggered breaths with spontaneous breaths allowed in between.

30. $\dot{V}_A$: Alveolar ventilation. $\dot{V}_A = (V_T - V_D)$ RR.

31. $\dot{V}_E$: minute ventilation. $\dot{V}_E = V_T$ x RR. Normal range is 5-8L/min.

32. **SaO$_2$:** Oxygen saturation: The percentage of all the available heme binding sites saturated with oxygen in the arterial blood.

33. **Tidal volume (V_T):** is the lung volume representing the normal volume of air moved into and out of the lung during one respiratory cycle. Normal range is 5-8ml/kg of ideal body weight.

Chapter 33 **References**

General References

1. MacIntyre NR. Mechanical Ventilation. Pennsylvania: WB Saunders, 2001.

2. Hess DR, Kacmarek RM. Essentials of Mechanical Ventilation, 2nd ed. New York: McGraw-Hill, 2002.

3. MacIntyre NR. Mechanical ventilation, 2nd ed. Missouri: Saunders Elsevier, 2009.

4. Tobin MJ. Principles and Practice of Mechanical Ventilation, 2nd ed. New York: McGraw-Hill, 2006.

5. Mackenzie I. Core Topics in Mechanical Ventilation. Cambridge, UK: Cambridge University Press, 2008.

Chapter references

1. Gonzalez M. Airway pressure release ventilation versus assist-control ventilation: a comparative propensity score and international cohort study. Intensive Care Med 2010; 36: 817-827. (Chapter 11)

2. Maxwell RA. A randomized prospective trial of airway pressure release ventilation and low tidal volume ventilation in adult trauma patients with acute respiratory failure. J Trauma 2010; 69: 501-10. (Chapter 11)

3. Taccone P. Prone positioning in patients with moderate and severe acute respiratory distress syndrome: a randomized controlled trial. JAMA 2009; 302: 1977-84. (Chapter 12)

4. Taylor RW. Low-dose inhaled nitric oxide in patients with acute lung injury: a randomized controlled trial. JAMA 2004; 13:1603-9. (Chapter 12)

5. Bollen CW. High frequency oscillatory ventilation compared with conventional mechanical ventilation in adult respiratory distress syndrome: a randomized controlled trial. Crit Care 2005; 4: R430-9. (Chapter 12)

6. Meade MO. Ventilation strategy using low tidal volumes, recruitment maneuvers, and a high positive end-respiratory pressure for acute lung injury and acute respiratory distress syndrome. JAMA 2008; 299: 637-645. (Chapter 12)

7. Lexi-comp Online Drug reference. http://www.crlonline.com/crlsql/servlet/crlonline Accessed on 2 Dec 2010. (Chapter 20)

8. Jacobi J, Fraser GL, Coursin DB. Clinical Practice Guidelines for the Sustained Use of Sedatives and Analgesics in the Critically Ill Adult. Crit Care Med 2002; 30:119-41. (Chapter 20)

9. Hess DR, MacIntyre NR, Mishoe SC, Galvin WF, Adams AB, Saposnick AB. Respiratory Care Principles and Practice. Pennsylvania: WB Saunders, 2002. (Chapter 6)

10. Kacmarek RM. Ventilatory Adjuncts. Respiratory Care 2002; 47: 319-330. (Chapter 6)

11. MacIntyre NR. Mechanical Ventilation. Pennsylvania: WB Saunders, 2001. (Chapter 6)

12. Pisani MA, Kong SY, Kasl SV, et al. Days of delirium are associated with 1-year mortality in an older intensive care unit population. *Am J Respir Crit Care Med* 2009; 180:1092-7. (Chapter 28)

13. Davydow DS, Katon WJ, Zatzick ZF. Psychiatric morbidity and functional impairments in survivors of burns, traumatic injuries, and ICU stays for other critical illnesses: a review of the literature. Int Rev Psychiatry. 2009; 21:531-8. (Chapter 28)

14. Kapfhammer HP, Rothenhausler HB, Krauseneck T, et al. Posttraumatic stress disorder and health-related quality of life in long-term survivors of acute respiratory distress syndrome. Am J Psychiatry 2004; 161:45-52. (Chapter 28)

15. Atabai K, Matthay MA. The pulmonary physician in critical care 5: Acute lung injury and the acute respiratory distress syndrome: definitions and epidemiology. Thorax 2002; 57: 452-458. (Appendix)

16. Fartoukh M, Maître B, Honoré S, Cerf C, Zahar J, Brun-Buisson Cl. Diagnosing pneumonia during mechanical ventilation-the clinical pneumonia infection score revisited. American Journal of Respiratory and Critical Care Medicine 2003; 168; 173-179. (Appendix)

Table 1: Calculation of the lung injury score

Table 2: The modified clinical pulmonary infection score

Table 3: Important numbers

Table 4: Useful Formulas

TABLE 1: Calculation of the lung injury score

	Score
Chest radiograph	
No alveolar consolidation	0
Alveolar consolidation confined to 1 quadrant	1
Alveolar consolidation confined to 2 quadrants	2
Alveolar consolidation confined to 3 quadrants	3
Alveolar consolidation confined to 4 quadrants	4
Hypoxemia score	
PaO_2/FiO_2 ≥300	0
PAO_2/FiO_2 225–299	1
PaO_2/FiO_2 175–224	2
PaO_2/FiO_2 100–174	3
PaO_2/FiO_2 <100	4
PEEP score (when mechanically ventilated)	
≤5 cm H_2O	0
6–8 cm H_2O	1
9–11 cm H_2O	2
12–14 cm H_2O	3
≥15 cm H_2O	4
Respiratory system compliance score (when available)	
≥80 ml/cm H_2O	0
60–79 ml/cm H_2O	1
40–59 ml/cm H_2O	2
20–39 ml/cm H_2O	3
≤19 ml/cm H_2O	4
The score is calculated by adding the sum of each component and dividing by the number of components used.	
No lung injury	0
Mild to moderate lung injury	0.1–2.5
Severe lung injury (ARDS)	>2.5

TABLE 2: The modified clinical pulmonary infection score

CPIS Points	0	1	2
Tracheal secretions	Rare	Abundant	Abundant + purulent
Chest X-ray infiltrates	No infiltrate	Diffuse	Localized
Temperature, °C	≥36.5 and ≤38.4	≥38.5 and ≤38.9	≥39 or ≤36
Leukocytes count, per mm^3	≥4,000 and ≤11,000	< 4,000 or > 11,000	< 4,000 or > 11,000 + band forms ≥500
PA_{O2}/FI_{O2}, mm Hg	> 240 or ARDS		≤240 and no evidence of ARDS
Microbiology	Negative		Positive

Definition of abbreviations: ARDS = acute respiratory distress syndrome; CPIS = clinical pulmonary infection score.

The modified CPIS at baseline was calculated from the first five variables. The CPIS gram and CPIS culture were calculated from the CPIS baseline score by adding two more points when gram stains or culture were positive. A score of more than six at baseline or after incorporating the gram stains (CPIS gram) or culture (CPIS culture) results was considered suggestive of pneumonia. Reprinted with permission of the American Thoracic Society. Copyright © American Thoracic Society - see reference 16.

TABLE 3: Important numbers

Peak pressure	Should not exceed 40 cm H_2O
Plateau pressure	Should not exceed 30 cm H_2O
Cuff pressure	Should be keep < 20 cm H_2O
A-a gradient	<10 mmHg
Minute ventilation ($\dot{V}_E$)	5-8 L/min.
Static Compliance	>60 ml/cmH_2O
Dynamic Compliance	40-50 ml/cmH_2O
PaO$_2$ / FiO$_2$	Normal range is 350-450 mmHg ALI <300 mmHg ARDS <200mmHg
RSBI(rapid shallow breathing index)	≤ 105 breaths/liter
Negative inspiratory force (NIF)	More negative than - 20 cm H_2O
Forced vital capacity (FVC)	≥ 10 ml/kg of IBW.

TABLE 4: Useful Formulas

Ideal body weight (kg)	Males: = 52 + (1.85 x (h-60)) Females: = 49 + (1.65 x (h-60)) h (height) in inches
Minute ventilation ($\ddot{V}_E$)	V_T x RR
A-a gradient	$PAO_2 - PaO_2$
PAO_2	$PiO_2 - PACO_2/R \rightarrow$ $FiO_2(713)$ -($PACO_2$ x 1.25) mmHg
PiO_2	FiO_2 (Patm – 47 mm Hg). Where Patm is the atmospheric pressure (760 mmHg at sea level).
Static Compliance	V_{TE} /(Plateau pressure – PEEP)
Dynamic Compliance	V_{TE} /(Peak pressure – PEEP)
Alveolar ventilation	$(V_T - V_D)$ RR

Pagers and Phone numbers

Interesting cases